Life's Little Adventures: The Journey Home

Mark McGrath

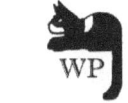

Whimsical Publications, LLC

Florida

Life's Little Adventures: The Journey Home is a work of non-fiction. Names, characters, and incidents are the products of the author's imagination and/or recollection and are either fictitious or are used fictitiously. Any resemblance to actual events or persons, living or dead, is entirely coincidental.

If you purchased this book without a cover, you should be aware that this book may have been stolen property and reported as "unsold and destroyed" to the publisher. In such case, neither the publisher nor the author has received payment for this "stripped book."

Copyright © 2009 by Mark McGrath
All rights reserved

No part of this book may be reproduced in any form or by any electronic or mechanical means, including information storage and retrieval systems, without prior written permission from the copyright holder and the publisher of this book, except by a reviewer who may quote brief passages in a review.

Published in the United States by
Whimsical Publications, LLC
Florida

http://www.whimsicalpublications.com

ISBN-13: 978-1-936167-04-3

Cover art by Janet Durbin
Editing by Krystal Cranfield

Printed in the United States of America

Dedication

Writing a dedication to a book that I never thought I would write is probably the most difficult task attached to this. What originally started out as nothing more than a series of essays and writings to friends about the trip from Florida to New York mushroomed rather quickly into stories about life and observations.

Writing anything isn't necessarily an easy task because the author has to think of his reader, his *audience,* and hope that the message or story he is trying to convey captures the imagination of those people who sit down and read it. I have always liked to write, but I can be a bit long winded, so sitting down and actually *doing* it was something that demanded commitment. I took on that task for the sake of those people I left behind in Florida in December of 2008.

Traveling that distance with the kids was a learning experience, and I could not have gotten custody of them without the help of someone who knew the legal system. She had the ability to relate her own experiences to me, and also the knowledge to help draft documents and navigate a twisted legal system. The commitment she showed to those tasks, even as she battled her own issues, was one of the driving factors that allowed me to fight as I should have and to eventually get the agreement signed.

Sometimes in the face of crisis it takes someone outside of the loop to bring me back to reality, and on many occasions she did. Thank you, Jodi.

I thank Pam Jones who was the *first* person who encouraged me to keep giving more and more, and to try to find a venue for the stories that I am driven to tell people. Having a small select group of friends allows me to talk directly to them and give more detail and more of the real me into the things that I write.

I thank all of those friends I reconnected with, and the ones I didn't know *before* I started this. They asked for and encouraged me to write more and to pursue something that I never thought I could do. The internet is a wonderful tool and it allowed me to seek and find people I had lost, and in turn those people connected me to a whole variety of new friends. If it weren't for the encouragement of *all* of those involved (there are *so* many to name and it would be grossly unfair to exclude any, so please forgive me if I can't include a list), *none* of these words would be read other than by me.

A special heartfelt thank you to Patrice who took time out of a long, busy schedule to edit the first piece of mine that was published (and included in its entirety here), and telling me, a fledgling writer at best, that she thought as a professional writer herself, that maybe I had something here and to keep going. Thank you to Margaret, a lost friend from high school years, who re-connected and gave me the incentive to seek people out to guide me in improving my writing.

Thank you to the long list of Facebook friends who *asked* for more even when I thought I couldn't do this. Thank you Amanda, the person directly responsible for leading me to Janet, who read a half-assed, unedited file of stories I had and said to me, "I will publish it when you are done."

Thank you to my parents. Although apart now and not on the best of terms, they taught me that with enough hard work *anything* is possible.

To mom who took us into her small place in Bayside and helped with the kids every single day. Without you things would be hectic and unsettled and I am thankful every day that you are there for them.

Thank you to my extended family (my ex's parents and sisters); without their support of the children and my effort to bring them back to New York, we never would have gotten out. And thank you to my ex, the mother of the kids who did a great deed and performed a selfless act by signing the custody papers and allowing the kids to leave Florida and come home.

My children are the reason I wake up in the morning and continue my work as an RN even on those days when I feel I have nothing left. They are the sole reason that anything for me exists, and I wrote this for them. One day many years after I am gone and they are in a library, they can take this eclectic mix of things daddy did and wrote about and show my great grandchildren what I left behind.

A special thank you to my sister Kelly and her husband Billy for years of support and helping with the kids. And to

Alice, Natalie and Mr. Kaplan who without hesitation allowed me to come back to work for a small family-like company. You *can* go home again, and they helped prove it.

To all of my family, my brothers, aunts, uncles and cousins, your support and unwavering love for the kids made the long, arduous journey home worth it.

To all my colleagues, friends and co-workers in Florida: I miss you all and not a day goes by where I don't have you in my thoughts. Thank you for affording me the opportunity to get to know and work with each and every one of you.

I humbly dedicate this book of stories to all of you.

Life's Little Adventures: The Road Home

TABLE OF CONTENTS

The Long and Winding Road...	Pg 1
The Best Laid Plans of Mice and Men	Pg 5
An Arctic Welcome Home...and Stuck in a Glacier	Pg 11
Santa Claus is Really Me in a Red Suit.	Pg 15
Art...and Elvis on Velvet	Pg 21
Heroes...and Daddy	Pg 26
What Happens in an Instant?	Pg 35
For Mischa...	Pg 43
Executive Decisions and Puppies	Pg 55
Great Grandma, Revenge and Spooks	Pg 62
Death Isn't the Worst Thing	Pg 71
Sometimes You Learn to Duck	Pg 81
It Happens When You Least Expect It	Pg 88
Memories of Time Past	Pg 98
DNR	Pg 110
Watch Your Speed	Pg 119
You Always Remember Your First...	Pg 128

LOOK AT ME, DADDY	Pg 137
Why is the Closet Closed?	Pg 143
The End?	Pg 148

The Long and Winding Road...

With all due respect to the Beatles, I chose this as the title to simply state that the road *home* was both long, winding and full of plot twists and adventures. Quite possibly it was the most exciting trip I have ever been on, and one I will never forget. This is the story of our trip *home*.

The U-Haul was packed, our lives crammed into cardboard boxes and plastic bins, and when you get right down to it, it's amazing that you can look at the lives of five people compacted into such a small amount of space. I often joked with friends and co-workers about taking the kids on a rambling twelve state killing spree (Okay, it was more like ten, but who really cares at this point?), and though no real people were actually killed, the destruction and carnage left behind us will be remembered by all for years to come.

We left at 11:30 a.m. on December 18th, my dad behind me in the U-Haul, and I was in the car (a Mazda RX 8, easily fast, but not a practical *daddy* car), and we hit the road for what seemed like a smooth ride. The little boys were in the back watching Horton (and I *highly* recommend portable DVD players, thank you Ja *HE SUS*!!!!!) and Julia sat with her American Girl doll, chatting away as Daddy navigated Interstate 95.

We got out of Florida rather quickly, and soon after crossing the Georgia border we stopped for some much needed rest. The kids expelled their gas, I filled the tanks and we left again with a bag of peaches, some boiled peanuts and a bumper sticker that said, "I ate a PEACH in Georgia...Come again soon!"

The kids didn't get it, and Dad just rolled his eyes.

Along the way, the kids kept asking are we *there yet*? All those years ago I remember fondly driving in my dad's old green station wagon to the Jersey shore and hearing him say, "*Yes, we are*! You can jump now." Trips in the car with my parents and my sister Kelly were always long, but, in the end, the time we spent together on the beach in New Jersey is something that I haven't forgotten even though some thirty years have passed since we last made that trip as a family.

We raced out of Georgia (OK, Dad was doing like fifty-five, and I was screaming internally for him to drive faster hoping that I didn't pop an aneurysm and have to have surgery in rebel country). I did pass a few hitchhikers along the way, but rather than pick them up thought to myself, "now where the *fuck* am I going to tie this numbskull to the car?" It's not as if I had *any room* for them, and I was a Yankee in rebel territory.

I was rather nervous being a true Yankee, you know, being in the *South* and all. I had never quite gotten used to seeing rebel flags and the different type of lifestyle, and I had always considered myself to be a New Yorker.

As the sun started to set and the temperature dropped, we stopped to eat at a Bo Jangles Chicken place. The kids filled up on chicken, biscuits and the trimmings.

So much for their last meal in the Deep South!

We left the gas station/rest stop/whatever the fuck it was called place and decided that the best place to stop was at that Bastion of Capitalism, *South of the Border*! I had been there once on our trip down seven years prior, and forgot what a real cheese factory it was. Bright neon signs and tourist traps lit the darkness in startling reds and blues, and I thought to myself...this *Pedro* guy has some racket going.

There was one thing though. Except for a drug store, which, by the way, doubled as a bathroom *and* a fireworks factory, everything was *closed*. The neon flashed, but *nothing* was to be had. I was kind of disappointed in a way. Here we were on a mad dash North and *no* one was there to greet us, wish us well or even offer a fucking Welcome to South of the Border. I was annoyed that not much was open, but I did step into the drug store with the kids in tow and what did I do?

I bought a few cheap souvenirs (mine was a XX sized T shirt that said: I made PEDRO MY BITCH at SOUTH OF THE BORDER), some snacks and drinks for the kids along with a beer for Dad and we headed to the first place local to bed down for the night.

One good thing about my dad being sixty-six now: he

gets all these *great* discounts! When we stopped at a Motel 8 and got a room for the night, we got exactly $4.55 off the bill. We headed for room 110, tired and bleary eyed from the trip. Both dad and I were exhausted from driving and the kids needed some time to unwind as well. I was relieved to see a door in front of me with a bed beyond it beckoning us to sleep.

I tried the door numerous times with no success, inserting the keycard five times and I kept getting a red light. Now, that was odd. I had just paid a whole $40.45 for the room and wanted nothing more than a pillow under my head. Dad, in his infinite wisdom, said, "You're doing it wrong." And, of course being the respectful son I am, I said, "Okay wise ass, you try." He promptly did and much to his embarrassment met with the same futile results.

As the two of us and the four now frustrated kids stood there dumfounded, the door opened and an angry voice screamed, "*We are in here. The asshole at the desk rented this already!*" The genius at the front desk somehow *forgot* to enter into his ancient computer that he had previously rented the room. Mea Culpas followed.

I thought to myself that the girl in the room with him was probably more pissed off then he was. I did hear her say, "What moron rents a room *twice*?", and I decided I had to act. The simple answer I wanted to say was, "Well obviously Skippy at the front desk of this paradise did." But somehow I thought better of it and simply walked away and made my way back to the office.

A few minutes later, and after having to hear some lame excuse as to *how* the past scene happened, I was given the key to another room. Room 111. Immediately next to *theirs*! I decided that I had to do *something* to make up for interrupting what was *obviously* another couple *sleeping*. I returned to the office, went into the bathroom and got them a gift.

And suffice it to say, The Trojan Rubber Company is exactly two dollars richer these days thanks to the contribution of one Mark A McGrath.

I left the gift in the door for them, although I am not sure if it was actually used. No matter though, it truly is the thought that counts and after all, isn't it *my job* as a nurse to prevent the spread of AIDS and STD's?

Quite frankly, I thought it was hilarious!

When I came back into the room laughing quietly under my breath, I told the kids that the people next door were playing volleyball and if they heard any noise to ignore it. I also told them that if it sounded like someone was moaning it meant that they hit the wall too hard and were hurt. Julia asked me if I would go help them if anyone got hurt because I was a nurse, and maybe "that was a good thing to do?" I told her that if it was an all girl team I would be more than happy to go over, but not to worry, Daddy wasn't needed there. Too bad for me!

My dad spit his drink out in a fit of laughter and just shook his head as he normally does when I become the wise ass I always seem to be. I love the innocence of my daughter. She gave me a bewildered look and went to brush her teeth.

We bedded down fast, and I don't recall if there was any noise. If there was, since I wasn't involved, I really didn't care much. I drifted off into a soundless, deep sleep and dreamt of home.

The Best Laid Plans of Mice and Men

Steinbeck had it right. The Best Laid plans of Mice and Men are often torn asunder, cast aside and changed as life throws curveball after curveball. Our second day was no exception, but it started out rather quiet and mundane.

The kids awoke at 6:45 a.m., hungry and wanting to get to New York, all the while thinking that four more hours was all we had left to go. I had to explain to them that there was four hours to go to the *border* of the next state! Packing them up was easy since I didn't take anything out of the car other than a handheld duffle with a quick change of clothes. We retired to the spacious dining area for a wonderful array of powdered donuts, cereals, and decaf coffee for Dad, and sat down for what was a quick sugar load for the kids.

Alex decided that he should have the Fruit Loops and proceeded to hand feed himself one at a time from the dispenser. I explained as best I could *why* he shouldn't put his hands in the jar. In his own affable way he said to me, "I know what to do, Daddy. I only want the blue ones."

Hard to argue with that logic, I suppose, and I watched as he only took the blue ones: *one at a time*. I have found out the hard way that arguing with Alex is a little like shooting an elephant with a squirrel gun. Basically, it is completely useless.

We left after making sure our neighbors were safe in room 110 (the Trojan was off the door, and I smiled at my good deed for the decade), and I loaded the little boys and Julia with me, and Jon climbed into the U-Haul with dad.

We hit I-95 at roughly eight am after a quick stop across the street for gas and snacks. As soon as everything was paid for, it was off to the races yet again.

The drive wasn't so bad for the first few hours; the temperature dropped a bit as we went north. Dad and I kept up a steady 65 mph on the highway and really, the Carolinas brought us nothing more than a long boring drive. I watched the road signs and the miles peel off and soon the trees were changing from Palms to hardwoods. Soon it became overcast and gray and a light rain began to fall.

Now you might think the ride was *boring*, with Alex and Aidan were in the back seat, *quiet* as mice watching the portable DVD. About one quarter of the way into Virginia I remarked, "Alex...if I have to hear Horton *one more time*...I will do a Van Gogh on myself and scream so loud I will *hear it*!"

His answer was a simple sentence, "I watching Horton, Daddy...you weird."

Again my son knew me, and it was hard to argue with him. Besides, arguing with him was a bit like hearing Horton Hears A Who ten times in a row. After a while I realized you can't argue with an eight year old, and that it was better to cut your losses knowing that Horton was a tad schizophrenic. I thought to myself, if he kept my kids entertained, well then, who the hell was I to argue?

Personally, I think Dr. Seuss suffered from the affliction. I mean, talking elephants in the land of WHO? Certainly Van Gogh had it; he cut his ear off to make the voices go away. Me? I'd have no such luck because if I cut *both* ears off I'd still hear that fat bastard elephant in my head telling the world that *Whoville* was in the little dust speck he held.

So much for my hallucinations and thank you Horton, for bringing them about yet again.

I did, however, get to hear all of the lost Scooby Doo episodes as well, from a childhood long since gone. Julia was quiet as she watched her DVD, and I thought....*SCOOBY DOO!* I love that show and pound for pound, he was one of our finest American actors.

The rain began to fall harder and more steadily, increasing in intensity through the lower part of Virginia. The drive got slower as the rain beat a steady rhythm on the windshield. I grew concerned when I no longer saw Dad in the rearview mirror. As my phone rang I said, "Yeah, Dad?" All I heard was, "Blowout, turn around now."

I got off at the next exit, doubled back onto the Southbound thruway and saw our little U-Haul on Northbound 95, crippled on the side of the road. The rain was pouring down hard and I had to pull over on a wet, sloppy shoulder so I could help Dad. My concern was with a truck losing control and plowing into us, so I wanted to get the kids off the road safely as fast as I could.

Dad had made the call to the U-Haul roadside service while I was getting to him. He was told he had to wait until he got a call back. The rain was driving and the cold, biting wind made it colder than it needed to be. Jon was scared and I could understand why. The rear passenger tire was a mess of twisted rubber, and I thought that it was a miracle they got off the road as they did.

Since Dad wasn't *supposed* to be driving the U-haul, I put Jon into my car with the other kids and gave him the go ahead to take them to lunch at the next exit. I would wait for the roadside service.

Dad chose the Waffle House because we could see the sign a little further ahead and it seemed like as good a place as any to feed the four kids. Besides, when we asked them where they wanted to eat, Alex saw the sign and said, "I want waffles." The screams from all four of them made the decision a rather easy one.

He left around 1 p.m., my kids safe with their grandpa for what we hoped would be a quick lunch. I watched as he slowly took my *sports* car back onto the highway and finally figured out that if he actually pushed the accelerator, the car would go faster. They soon disappeared into the rainy day, and I retired to the truck to wait for the new tire.

Shortly after 3 p.m., a truck pulled up behind me. The tow truck driver was there, ready to change the tire. I noted the Confederate Flag and the SOUTH SHALL RISE AGAIN bumper sticker and smartly decided now was *not* the time to say that they got their asses kicked in the war and to *get over it*.

I was his faithful Sancho Panza, driving the truck onto a block of wood so he could change the tire.

Right around 4 pm, I was on the road again: cold, miserable and thankful that the kids were safe and terrorizing the Waffle House staff. I don't think that the staff at this particular Waffle House will ever be the same again, especially after two hours of the four McGrath kids asking questions and making a racket.

We gassed again, got back on the road, and I don't care *what* pilots tell you, you *cannot* make up time on the road or in the air. I always thought that was the dumbest thing I ever heard but we tried to pick up speed through Virginia.

We ran into what was a parking lot on 95 as we got closer to the bigger cities and the lower DC area. We were able to meander our way along the I-95 corridor slowly, and through a pounding rain. I had been getting weather updates from home; we were heading into the first real snow of the year.

Wonderful, just fucking wonderful.

As it got darker and the traffic was heavy, I decided to look at my bank accounts to make sure the endless drain on the money was still steady. As I looked, I was not only pissed off, but I wondered if I was going to have to turn around and admit myself to Parrish Medical Center's (my now previous place of employment) Stroke Center with a bleed: 1,700 dollars was missing!

I called Bank of America and they promptly told me that the check my asswipe ex-landlord gave me *bounced*. I called him and did my best to remain as calm as I possibly could (which was *no* small feat, and one that anyone who knows me will agree was virtually impossible). I got a cock and bull story about how I was *supposed* to paint and blah, blah, blah, and he said he put a stop payment on it. I called the bank again, and was told it bounced.

Needless to say, by the time Dad found me screaming my lungs out at the landlord, sending the locals scrambling like ants for cover, and ready to pop a blood vessel, I was ready to go on a *one* state killing spree.

Straight to New Jersey. The fucker robbed me.

I called my ex-wife's sister, a prominent attorney in Albany who as always, calmed me down and told me it would be taken care of. I told her, it sure would, I was stopping in Jersey in person to extract my money in flesh. However, cooler heads prevailed (not mine, but what the *fuck* did you expect? 1,700 dollars gone in a flash), and I decided to let the matter drop until such time as I was able to get to court to screw him and his dad out of 6K. You see, the Florida laws allow for three times the damages and fees.

So, really, you know who you guys are...*fuck you*. Your time will come.

After making a scene as only I can, and after a quick potty break at a small roadside rest stop, which was now full of trucks and bleary eyed drivers, four kids and a crazed

Bronx Irishman, we set off yet again.

The weather was getting worse and the cold was beginning to bite harder. At that particular point something occurred to me. Wearing crocs with no socks was probably pretty dumb. No matter, though. I couldn't really feel my feet anyway, and the cold wakes me up more.

We raced through DC, and as we passed Camden Yards, I casually flipped the bird at the Orioles home park. We gathered speed and made excellent time after that. We stopped one more time for gas in Delaware, feeding the kids road kill sandwiches and Oreos, and raced as fast as we could through Southern NJ and up to the Turnpike.

All was well right until we got to Newark; then ice, snow and a lovely northern snow storm was what we had to drive through. Welcome back guys!

We got to the airport exit at 10 p.m. and it seemed as if no one except us was on the road. The snow was falling steadily and the icy roads made for a challenging drive to the bridge. I crept slowly toward the toll plaza at the exit to the George Washington Bridge, and as the snow and ice pelted the car I realized one thing.

We were close. So close in fact that I could see parts of the city through the snow and haze. It was then that it finally hit me...

We were *home*.

I often wondered what ruby slippers could really do. I found out when I saw my city that night with frozen tears stuck to my cheeks.

Don't ever leave home, gang. Because when you do and you need to go back, the sadness at what and who you leave behind is heartbreaking. Fixing a broken heart is difficult, even for good nurses and doctors.

The last miles on the road clicked by slowly as the car slid across the icy roads into the Bronx. We crawled like a snail along the Cross Bronx Expressway and onto the last thing that separated us from finally being home.

The Whitestone Bridge stood before us, and as I paid the final toll and began the slow painful drive across I could feel the knot in my stomach turn tighter. We crossed and drove the last mile and a half; I realized that my grip on the wheel was tight and I was sweating from being nervous.

We got to moms' at 11:55 p.m., with the kids wide

awake and hungry, asking for dinner.

It was like we had never left.

They sat down to a hearty meal made long before and now reheated by NaNa, and I sat on the couch and closed my eyes, weary from the long drive.

An Arctic Welcome Home...and Stuck in a Glacier

Thousands of years ago Horton's great hairy ancestor, the great wooly mammoth, trudged across frozen glaciers in what was the last great ice age in history.

Or so I thought.

I often read up on topics of interest, mostly science stuff, and mostly historical science at that. Fat wooly Hortons are often found buried and preserved in areas once covered by huge expanses of permafrost. As the Earth heats up because of what some people call Global Warming, the preserved Uncles of Horton are revealed, giving us a look into the not so distant past. After hearing that movie the whole way home, I say good for you, hairy bastards. You got what you deserve and it serves you right for dumping a fat, dopey, talking elephant into my psychosis.

On the other hand it makes me think of how fucking cold a northern storm can be. And what a colossal pain in the ass it is to have to try and dig your way out. Now for most of you, my faithful readers, it's pretty easy. You live north and can relate. Me? What was I thinking when all I had on was summer shoes, no socks and a flimsy jacket to protect me from the elements? I suppose it serves me right for leaving in the beginning of winter.

The U-Haul was encased in snow and ice, and my nice Mazda RX 8 was in its own frozen tomb, much like good ole Horton's long dead hairy uncle. The good thing was that both batteries had a good charge and both cars started easily. The bad thing was that neither had tires suitable for navigating and driving on ice, and as I tried to force the Mazda out, I managed to spin in a 360 and face oncoming traffic.

And I'm supposed to be smart.

I tried in a futile attempt to free the car from the ice, but the only luck I had was managing to spin completely around and face the opposite direction. Back and forth I rocked the car, and after a half hour and with three teenagers pushing, I managed to skid the car back into the frozen tomb it started from.

I unloaded the U-Haul one box and bin at a time, and by the time I had made 5 trips back and forth, I was thinking...you know...if I had that fat bastard Horton here right now, I could load up his back and we could do this all in one fell swoop. Or, he could just pull the cars out of the iceberg.

It was about then that I realized my meds weren't working anymore, because here I was a perfectly sane forty-three year old father of four kids stuck in ice, muttering about some fat bastard elephant named Horton and why wasn't he there pulling my sorry ass out of the ice?

I went back and promptly took the DVD out of the car, buried it in a box and stored it in the attic. I kept hearing Horton's voice and I was hoping that by storing the DVD in a place far from me, the talking elephant would finally go away.

It began to rain and that really made unloading harder. My sister showed up with her two children and she and Mom prepped for what was to be a big soiree at Trudy's place. The truth of the matter was that I had it easy. All I needed to do was walk through slush, and have my feet freeze off because I refused to wear socks and was still wearing crocs. They, on the other hand, were dealing with six kids and preparing all the food. I guess I am pretty smart after all.

Trudging through the muck really wasn't all that bad. Considering the size of the place we moved to, the cold wasn't so bad after all. I did manage to get to the grocery store and I oriented myself to the shopping center behind the apartment. Still it was cold and I was wishing for some warmer shoes. I did try one place but having size fourteen feet makes getting shoes a task, and when they told me the shoes could be ordered, I uttered a quick no thanks and went back home.

The official welcome home was December 21st when my sister and I took *all six kids* into New York City to see the Radio City Christmas Spectacular. We decided it was best to each take the train to Penn Station, meet there, and then train it to Radio City rather than drive into the city in the middle of the Christmas rush. Indeed that turned out to be the smartest decision made on this whole fantastic voyage.

The kids and I started out on the bus. We walked in the cold and then stood idly by as cars passed us while we waited for the Q13 to show up. Once the bus came and we got on, the driver said, "Pay two fares only," and I thought, hey, what a *bargain* for me! We exited to dropping temperatures and wind, and I bought tickets on the LIRR and a Metro card for the return home.

The LIRR train came and the kids struck up a conversation with the conductor, asking him his name, where he was from and did he like punching tickets. The 50,000 dollar question was, you guessed it, "Are we in New York City yet, daddy?" I told them time after time that when we go through the tunnel, the train stops and we all get out, then we will be in New York.

We made it in no time as stop after stop whizzed by much like the last twenty years of my life. When we did make it to Penn, I took a few pictures of the kids near the ticket booth and Christmas tree. Jon was somewhat upset by the two homeless guys he saw, and asked, "How does one become homeless?"

From the mouths of babes, faithful readers; the question couldn't be answered right no matter what I said. So I simply told him, "I dunno, Jon, maybe he lost his job and can't get a new one?" Jon in his infinite wisdom says, "Well, why can't he just get a new one?"

Again, very hard to answer correctly and I didn't want to give Jon a dissertation on the plight of the homeless.

We met my sister Kelly and the kids, and I must say the kids were adorable. The funniest part of the day happened as the Uptown 1 train was thundering down the tracks headed toward our stop. Six kids, a cranky-assed daddy and my pregnant sister in the midst of holiday shoppers miserable for various reasons, but mostly because the train was packed like the proverbial sardine can.

There we are trying to maintain sanity and this homeless lady (or rather she appeared as one...I still debate it, much like what was that stuff I cleaned out of my fridge before I left? Could be cheese; could be a new life form, I'm not sure; who the fuck knows.). Anyway, she is pushing her way through the crowd and says, I *shit you not*, "Can anyone spare some change for a grilled cheese sandwich? The deli closes in an hour so I need it now!"

Now *that* takes balls, kids, and mighty big ones at that. When she got to me, I handed her a buck. My sister looked at me cross-eyed as I told the lady, "Look, here's a buck. Get to the deli, and tell the deli guy to throw on a slice of tomato as well. I want my buck's worth!" The guy sitting next to Jon looks at me like I'm some tourist schmuck and I said to him flatly, "Look, I've heard every excuse; that was the best one! The deli is closing in an hour. Shit, I should have tossed her a five and told her to get fries, too!"

My sister smacked me in the head as we exited to 50th Street.

The city was alive at night. Street vendors sold knock off purses, the kind my friend Brittany constantly covets. Gucci, Fendi, you name it, you can get it all in one long winding city block. I could smell the charcoal cooking the pretzels and chestnuts. Thousands of New Yorkers rushed about as the eight of us made our way to Radio City. The air was crisp, dry and steam rose out of the manhole covers like mist on a lake in the early spring. We made our way to the line and entered the hallowed halls of Radio City.

The kids were excited. I was excited because well...the Rockettes are pretty hot and all those legs dancing in a line seemed like it would be worth every penny I paid for the tickets.

And two hours later, when it was over, it was worth it.

My kids thanked me for the best Christmas gift *ever*. The smile I cracked was the biggest one I had in such a long time. I yearned for home for so long and now I was here.

Whoever said you can't go home again was full of shit. I think it was Horton, but that dumb bastard is still stuck with his ball of dust and Whoville. I have it much better.

I have my kids and my city, and really, is there anything else I can ask for?

I suppose there is one thing more I can ask for but I'll get to that later.

Santa Claus is Really Me in a Red Suit.

If you sit down and think about how things turn out, you realize that no matter how hard you try, control is one thing that none of us really has. Take my friend Horton for instance. Logically speaking, no sane talking elephant would ever tell anyone about a world living in a speck of dust now, would he?

He had total control over *everything* and look where that got him. It got him thrown into a box and stored in the attic in a DVD case along with old books and DVD's that are not of the family variety. Controlling your own destiny, Horton, my dear friend, is something you should have concentrated on harder instead of trying to drive me completely out of my mind.

Anyway, Christmas Eve was creeping around the bend, and the family was going to bombard my poor mom's small apartment for a feast! The one food I missed most while I was gone was mom's lasagna. Now we all know with a name like McGrath, no Italian exists in me *at all*.

However, as luck would have it, grandma married what passes for an Italian (he has the name, but that's about it, kids), and she was taught how to make it the *right* way. She then taught my mom.

Which, faithful reader, only benefits me. I ate lasagna in a bunch of places in Florida, and I can say that not *one* comes remotely close to either mom's or grandma's. So, coming home served at least one other purpose. And that was to eat some good home cooking and enjoying myself as I did.

The kids have this way of asking the same question 100 times, and the one resonating in my head was this, "Are you Santa Claus, Daddy?" Ha! My immediate thought was to just say the obvious, "Are you saying daddy is a big fat guy that slides down a chimney just to drop you gifts?" Or better yet, "Do I look like a damned Hallmark moment?" I thought better of it and simply answered, "Why would you ask such a silly question? Santa and I look nothing alike? How can Daddy be Santa Claus?"

Alex's simple answer was hysterical as he said, "You too skinny, Daddy, Santa fat!"

I simply smiled at the innocence of youth and thought to myself, *If I eat enough of that lasagna later, my ass will be fatter than Jolly Ole Saint Nick's!* I didn't have the heart to tell the two older ones that Santa is really a figurehead, and although years ago in a distant place a real Santa existed, nowadays he has been replaced by plastic figurines, Salvation Army workers ringing bells asking for donations, and the various esoteric traditional Christmas specials. I long for the days of my youth when I wished that Santa would bring me what I really wanted. This year, all I wanted was essentially what I already had: having my kids and a return to the home I left many years ago in a search for a life that I thought was better.

When you get down to brass tacks (I never quite got that saying because as far as this guy is concerned sitting on a brass tack leaves a bloody hole in your ass), I suppose that to each of us Christmas has a different meaning. If I use the kids as an example: at their ages now, the main idea of Christmas is getting as many things as they asked for from Santa. Kids don't necessarily get the whole idea behind Christmas, but I give them some latitude in their thinking.

As time marches on and progresses into wherever it takes us to in the end, the kids will see that Christmas is more than just about getting what you ask for. School and friends will eventually desensitize and sanitize their minds of any thoughts of a real Santa. I suppose that when he actually was *alive*, the real Mr. Claus (most likely German, the only Claus's I know all drink German Ale and eat Weiner schnitzel) started a tradition of giving gifts to friends once a year.

Now, we have giant department stores, Hallmark and a myriad of animated tales of Christmas to keep us going year after year. I still watch some of them; my favorite line is mimicked by Jerry Seinfeld. Hermie the Elf states, "But I don't wanna be an *elf* and make *toys*, I wanna be a dentist!" Seinfeld bit that line in the puffy shirt episode, "But I don't wanna be a pirate!" Again, so much for traditional Christmas

T.V. shows.

My favorite still has to be the one where we see a schizophrenic red nosed reindeer, Rudolf, flying with his cronies. Now personally the idea of reindeer pulling a fat guy in a sled over every roof in the world dropping sacks of toys and crap down chimneys is a bit hard to believe. But the kids seem to think that reindeer talk and a fat guy named Santa drops toys on them every year, so who the hell am I to argue with that?

Kids, I'll let you in a secret, your Daddy and family buy you all of your gifts. But daddy puts on a silly hat and eats the cookies each year, because, well, he loves you all. And the longer you believe in Santa, the tooth fairy and the Easter Bunny, the longer you will stay innocent and I can delay breaking reality to you.

Christmas, has so many meanings to so many different people, it's almost impossible to keep up anymore. I think for a lot of folks it's simply the spirit of giving things and feeling good about the end of the year and spending time with loved ones. I got my gift early by going to see the show with the kids and mom's lasagna.

For others, it's strictly a religious day. It's a day of reflection and celebration of a mythical birth date given to the Savior of humanity, Jesus Christ himself. Essentially, he was born in what amounted to be a stable full of animals and bedded down in a feeding trough. What's reality? If Mary and Joseph could only afford those accommodations, then, in my humble opinion, they did what they should have done. He started his life simply and died some thirty three or so years later.

Simplicity at its best, can anyone ask for anything more?

For me, the thing I wanted most was getting back home with my kids to the family I left behind seven years prior. I left a bunch of people in Florida that I love and care for, and that is always home number two for me. Leaving was hard, but the thing I wanted most was 1,215 miles away.

Before I left, I told a few people how I felt. I didn't reveal much to a few others because I was leaving and there was really no point.

I also got to think of the people I left here years ago, and then came back to. I got to see my mom's face when the kids finally came home for good and they got to see my dad, as well. Then seeing my ex-in-laws and how excited they were that we made it home and how much they missed the kids was worth everything as well.

Then I remembered my dear friend Michael, who died at thirty-eight from an insidious brain tumor and how it robbed him of his life and his family. And, then I thought about how his kids lost their daddy one week before Christmas and Hanukkah in 2005. I thought of how I doubted myself because I knew something was wrong months before he was diagnosed. I remember almost losing my own life and the lives of my then wife and two eldest kids in a horrible accident on the highway in 1998. That was December 26. I am home now, and I remember all that.

And so I cried, I laughed and I enjoyed the hell out of the first bite of mom's lasagna in seven long years.

You know what? It was still like I remembered: the best!

Christmas...home...my kids...and Horton the Elephant.

I'm never leaving again. You can always click your heels, but sometimes magic takes a while. Magic was the first night as we crossed the bridge in the driving snow, the car sliding at every twist and turn of the road. Magic was seeing mom and her tired, happy face as her grandkids made it back to the castle she calls her place in Queens. Magic was the day when their other grandparent's came and gave them all the winter clothes they could possibly need. Real magic was traveling back to the city, *our* city, and watching what was a great show at Radio City Music Hall.

Real Magic does exist. Sometimes if you wish hard enough, like Dorothy Gale in the Wizard of Oz, you can indeed get what you wish for. Wearing size fourteen ruby slippers makes walking extremely funny and often hurts, but the reality is, the more you wish and ask, the more likely you are to have me in a Red Suit drop your wish right in your lap.

So on Christmas my wish was realized when my sister and the kids, my two aunts and a few second cousins I hadn't seen in well, ever, came to Mom's and we dined. Outside it was cold and dreary, but I didn't want to dwell on the weather; having my family around me was just too important. My sister brought garlic mussels, which, by the way, were just ridiculously great. Her five year old son, Billy, dug through a bowl of them like a treasure hunter looking for gold. We had fine ravioli (the lasagna was for Christmas day!), clam dip and dessert, and to say it was all delicious wouldn't do it justice.

The kids got to open gifts with their cousins Billy and Gabby, and what a time was had by all of them! Paper flew off of neatly wrapped boxes each revealing its hidden treasure. There were Disney Cars toys for Alex, Star Wars toys for Aidan and an artist set for him as well. Jon got Star Wars collectibles and books, and Julia the Princess got collectible Barbie's. They also all got new clothes!

The *pièce de résistance* was the Wii we got Billy and Gabby. When they opened it, I didn't feel like the cheap prodigal uncle anymore. Both kids jumped on me and said thank you about a hundred times. The smile on all of the kids' faces was flawless, and worth everything it took to get back home.

We awoke on Christmas morning to our traditional eggs and bacon breakfast, a myriad of gifts, wrappings and batteries, and got dressed to head to my dad's and then to cousin Patty's for another round of fine American Cuisine. I dropped Mom off just before lunch, and headed to Dad's which much to her dismay was about a mile and a half from where Patty's house was. Mom and dad haven't been together in ten years and knowing that he lived close to where we were upset her.

I got to Dad's, he was smiling and looked weary, but happy we made it. My brother Cory was there lamenting over his new Rock Band game for the Xbox 360 because as is turned out...his was broken. Now he had to wait to play it. There was a Seinfeld game on the table and since he and I share such a cultish love of the show, we thought it would be interesting to see who knew more. Time was short, and although we wanted to sit and play, we deferred until we had enough time to devote to it.

I saw my brother, Sean, for the first time in three years; he was just as I remembered: outgoing, happy, and looking for his nephews and niece. Both of my brothers were as happy as dad and Leslie to see the kids, so our short stay flew by in a second. Then we were off to Patty's while dad and the rest went to brunch.

Patty's brought the same hilarity I remember. The house was warm, inviting, and I could smell food cooking (the lasagna was in the front of my mind). There was a huge tree (and it was male....there were a ton of balls on it), gifts and a nice warm fake fireplace creating just the right atmosphere. All we did was eat, watch Ice Age (HAHAHAHAHA!) and reminisce about those who died and weren't there to share the holiday.

We went home with the day's bounty firmly in the trunk, and I said to myself, "I missed this for eight Christmases?" Well, not anymore, gang. Not anymore.

I guess the moral of the story is that you can go home again. If the Wizard of Oz and Dorothy Gale teaches us anything it's this: With big enough wishes and large enough ruby slippers (in my case shoes!), you can get home again.

And for those that I left behind in my second home, I miss you all. It's not goodbye....it's see you soon!

I am a very, very fortunate man. And there really is a Santa Claus. I just wear a red suit once a year and stay in Holiday Inn Expresses just for the effect!

Art...and Elvis on Velvet

Someone once told me that art is what you see and how you interpret the object you are observing. Now, my idea of Art may be vastly different than a lot of people, so taking the kids to the Met the other day was an adventure to say the least. I didn't know what they would want to see, so I took it upon myself to show them the things I found to be art or items of interest from those periods in history that I found exciting.

Years ago, when I was about my eldest son's age, I can remember driving with my parents in the back of an old Kingswood Estate station wagon along various highways and byways in the Bronx, noticing just about anything on the road. I can remember driving past trucks that sold anything from one dollar watermelons to all types of "artwork." Plastic and carved wooden characters would often dot the road, for sale tags fluttering as people drove by flipping the bird or throwing half eaten cheeseburgers at the moron selling them.

It was then that I discovered velvet paintings. Very high on the art monitor they are, these portraits of Americana. Every summer we would see portraits of Sitting Bull, Christ, and my personal favorite, the King himself, one Elvis Aaron Presley. I used to ask my dad why we couldn't get a Day-Glo velvet painting of Elvis for the wall. His typical answer would be, "A velvet Elvis? Is that what you call art?"

No, but that wasn't the point, Daddyo. Now at forty-three and a dad myself, it was my job to explain what was art to the kids....velvet Elvis or no velvet Elvis.

I don't even like velvet...unlike George Costanza who would "drape himself in velvet..." I don't have any real use for it. The feel alone makes my skin crawl, so when I left the house early Tuesday my determination lead me to think historical rather than velvet art. I find paintings on cheap velvet to be rather cheesy, and I don't consider them to be real art. I have to admit, if I saw velvet paintings in the Met, I think I'd probably drop dead where I stood.

We took the bus again to the LIRR in the cold; the kids

were reminding me to watch the gap. Of course, Alex in his own repetitive way let everyone know at least fifty times to watch the gap or you'll die! I mean only a kid can put it so simply, yet so eloquently. I figured out that last time I ventured into the city with them that I had paid too much. Being the smart cheapskate I am, I bought one family ticket and we waited for the train. Once it came, we were on our way.

You might be asking yourself (then again maybe you aren't, but I'll ask the question for you, faithful reader), "What the fuck does a Velvet Elvis have to do with all of this?" Well, you'll see further on down the path. The kids were asking what they would see, and I said..."Well, *art* and things like that."

As the train rumbled on more questions came. They asked if any kids did the drawings and I almost laughed out loud. "No," I said simply, "all the people who did the pieces we are going to see are already dead."

Alex said, "When were they born, daddy. How old were they..." It was going to be a long visit. I could sense the excitement and anticipation in all of the kids.

We got off at Penn Station, and I called their Aunt Abby at the Met asking her advice on the best and fastest way to get to the museum. I decided to cab it, figuring the fifteen bucks it would cost would be worth it as the kids had never been in a yellow cab.

The city was gray and overcast. Busy. Steam wafted across the streets from the manholes and I could smell the bowels of the city in the air. A sea of yellow was outside Madison Square Garden, each cab waiting for a fare to take to any point in the city. We grabbed an SUV type car and piled in. Our driver, Ahknod, charged me an extra fare for all of us, and then took off to our destination on 5th Avenue.

I have to admit, I was never in a cab that had a touch screen in it. I was able to figure out that CNN was on, and at the touch of a finger you could see where you were going, how many people were hit along the way, and when poor Frogger was gonna get squished as he tried his best to dodge Ahknod the mad cabdriver.

A harrowing ten minutes dragged on and I think we drove on the sidewalk and took out a cafe and a hotdog vendor. I'm not really sure what happened...all I know is I kept my eyes shut, and the air smelled like mustard and sauerkraut as I handed Ahknod a twenty dollar bill and beat a hasty retreat to the confines of the Met and its treasures. The great thing about the trip was that the kids' aunt worked there, so admission was on the house.

We met Abby and rushed through the turnstiles and went straight to the Mummies. They liked the exhibit after all, though Aidan was dismayed to see an empty sarcophagus. I started to explain to him that they took the body out and used him as an extra in the latest version of the Mummy movie when a teacher who was giving a boring lecture on the fate of Egyptian antiquities to a bunch of snotty fourth graders shushed my kids.

Shushed.

Hmmm, I think a sarcastic remark was about to be said.

I let the kids and an obviously pissed off aunt move out of earshot as the kids from Mrs. Shush's' class gathered around the eight ton sarcophagus and began to listen to her explain about the container. Fifteen kids were standing there listening to Ms. Mary Jane Rotten Crotch, who stood under the open lid. I said aloud, "I'll give anyone twenty bucks to kick the lid closed." She shot me a look and said, "I am trying to teach, sir."

"Trying? Well, it seems to me that's all you're doing because no one here *gives a fuck* what you're saying. Maybe you should teach my kids who you told to be quiet."

Witch.

Anyway, I caught up with the kids in the room of armor and I have to tell you...I was smiling proudly at myself.

Medieval and Renaissance art is what I wanted to see, and the boys were interested in the variety of suits of armor and weapons available. I explained what a mace was, what a halberd did, and the various types of armor on display. Jon asked why anyone would wear a metal suit.

Fair question. My answer? I have no idea.

Jon said he thought I knew everything, and I firmly reminded him that if that's what the case actually was I would be shushing him in a room full of mummies and fourth graders.

The rolling eyes of a 12 year old... Priceless.

We stayed in that room for a bit and then headed to see invaluable paintings. I get overwhelmed at exhibits such as this, so I decided it was best to view more Renaissance paintings. As we went past the first guard I said to him, "Hey, do they have any paintings here of Elvis on velvet? I really wanna see one."

He looked at me and said, "No, sir. This is Renaissance art."

Even the guards have no sense of humor.

Elvis turned out to be much like the search for the Holy Grail...fruitless. Fun, but fruitless. If my brother Sean can see a sculpture of Michael Jackson and a chimp in the Louvre, why the fuck doesn't the Met have a velvet Elvis? I mean, it is art and, by the way, *I wanted to see one.*

No such luck, though.

I took a wealth of pictures and saw priceless works of art. Now if I were, say, Ferris Bueller (my idol. What a racket *that* guy had), I'd have taken the kids to a fancy place to eat and spent a couple of hundred bucks on pancreas, but since I didn't have the money, I thought the cafeteria was a better idea.

When I asked them there if they had pancreas, I thought that I'd be physically removed. One guy laughed when I said, "Look at my day! I have my four kids, took them in a cab, saw priceless works of art and damn if I want some pancreas!" He says to me, "Dude, I loved that movie!"

Yeah, so did I, but all I got was four orders of chicken nuggets which cost me $28.50.

We left Abby, who needed to return to work, and went and saw some Greek and Roman statues, which were nudes in case you didn't know. My Aidan let *everyone* know.

Aidan was standing next to a marble statue of Apollo and I said, "Aidan, let me take a picture of you there, smile." He runs away and yells, "Daddy, that statue has a penis on it, that's disgusting."

Well, hard to argue with him there, but nonetheless it was a priceless work done long ago and penis or *not*, I thought having my kid in a picture with a Roman god might be something nice to remember.

Julia says out loud, "Daddy, would *you* want to have someone take a picture of your penis?" At which point through fits of laughter from the surrounding peanut gallery, I ran for the exit.

I didn't stop laughing until we were out of the museum. We hopped on a bus back toward Penn Station. I wasn't paying Ahknod's brother, cousin or father a *dime* to drive us across town. The mustard from the first ride was still on my shirt. We got to Penn just in time to get on the last non-peak train back home, then on a bus, *et voila* (I hate French, except fries, and dressing, and well...), we were up the stairs and done!

Mom made it back shortly after and asked how the day was. As I was about to answer, Julia says," We saw paintings and mummies and plates and we ate in a cafeteria and a statue of a naked man and daddy wanted to see some guy named Elvis Velvet. Who is Elvis Velvet, Nana?"

Mom had no idea what that run-on sentence was about, but that night when I slept I dreamt George Costanza was draping me in velvet.

And Elvis was blasting on the radio.

Heroes...and Daddy

In the not so distant past and not long before we left Florida for good, Alexander was given an in school assignment on who he wanted to be like when he grew up. Since the age of two and a half, he has been given various diagnoses ranging from mentally retarded, autistic, PDD, hearing loss and everything in between.

Denial is one of those things we all experience at one time or another. I always knew something wasn't totally right with Alex, but I thought his hearing was the only issue and nothing else was wrong. When my former wife and I took him to a PhD for testing we were devastated.

An IQ of 54 will not function in society; he will need massive amounts of care and therapy and accordingly to her testing he was severely Autistic. I was told at the time that he might not speak and may never hold any kind of job.

Now, you can imagine just how unbearable it is to hear such news and then look into the big round face of your son, and hold it in your hands and cry as he stares blankly at you. You curse out loud and then, when all is said and done, when all the anger and sadness pours out of you like sand through a sieve, just when you think there is nothing more...

You sit on your couch when everyone is asleep, and you think. Think of what you'll have to do to help your child, you think of what it will take, and what it will cost in the end. You think of how your family and friends will be affected. All those thoughts race around inside the half empty echo chamber you call your skull, and you say to yourself *what am I going to do?*

The answer is plainly simple. You be Daddy. You be what your child needs. Daddy. And then when no one is looking, when the clan is fast asleep all tucked in and all you hear is the rhythmic breathing of your children, you look down at your son in your arms sound asleep, not a care in the world because you are his daddy and you're holding him.

You look down and you kiss his head and you say to him, "I love you Alex...everyone is wrong about you. Your future is bright and limitless."

When the moment comes and he turns and cuddles you, the floodgates open and you quietly cry yourself to sleep, protected by the person you are most worried about: your two and a half year old son.

I relate that story to you because all of it is true, and now, almost six years later, I can say that Alex is how I always describe him. He's Alex. He has his issues like most kids, and if I didn't say anything to tell you about who he is and why he does what he does, then you might look at him a little differently and just scratch your head. He isn't different, he is just my special boy, Alex. I call him special because that day the teacher called me into the office to show me his work, I knew what a gift I had.

His paper was simple, and his handwriting was legible for a change. The question the teacher asked her class was simple, yet very effective in eliciting a response. Who do you want to be like when you grown up, and why?

He wrote in his best print with very precise stokes: *I want to be like my daddy. He is a nurse. He saves people. He is my hero. I want to be a hero like daddy.*

I looked at the paper with a tear in my eye and said loud enough for his teacher Mrs. Lippert to hear, "No Alex you're wrong. I am not anything near a hero. My hero is *you*." We had a very quiet ride on the way home.

How do you begin to explain to a child what a hero is? I thought long and hard about how to put it into words. And I suppose no matter what I tell him, I don't actually have a concrete answer. I suppose when he reads this, he will have a better understanding of a plethora of things. And really, that is all I can ask as his dad.

Alex went through different tests: therapies for speech, behavior, fine and gross motor skills. I asked many people, doctor's, therapists, specialists, "Can my son hear me?" The answer was always *yes* from speech and language people, although I never believed it. I didn't care if one of the principal symptoms of Autism is not looking people in the eye or paying attention to them. When I took him to the hearing specialist and his hearing was tested in a controlled setting, do you know what the test showed?

Alex couldn't hear. I can't say it any plainer than that.

I remember asking the doctor, a brilliant man and very practical in his approach to things, "What should we do?" He simply stated that tubes in his ears would help drain all the fluid and make his eardrums work the way they were intended.

As was custom, I took Alex to the doctor that morning, and he sat and played with a puzzle as I read through an endless stream of fishing and old, tattered People magazines. The nurse led us into the exam room and while we waited for the doctor I looked at the tools he used and knew what some were for. Others were so archaic in design that I wondered silently what purpose they served.

The doctor came in with his usual lighted scope wrapped around his head and he said simply, "Alex will have surgery when you feel he is ready, and then we can start speech and language therapy."

"Do you think he can learn to talk?" I asked.

"Yes, he can. He can't learn what he can't hear. He'll need therapy and he may require it for years, but he'll talk."

I thanked him, paid the bill (which was worth every *dime* I spent, and one I happily paid), and we bolted home.

After telling his mother that the doctor had confirmed my suspicions, and knowing his speech therapist was coming over later in the day (we privately paid for therapy), I waited. I waited much like a deer hunter waits in a blind for his prey to come into sight, waiting for the exact moment before the trigger is pulled and then in a flash it's all over. When she came into the house, and began therapy, I walked into the room and without so much as a word out of my mouth I handed her the doctor's evaluation.

I turned and left, got my car keys and went for a drive. I didn't need to say anything, although inside I was a raging inferno. I had to dampen the flames, and there was too much fuel in my house.

So, instead of stoking the flames, I simply let them die down on their own. By the time I came home, she was gone, and Alex was playing in the play room just as he had been when I left him with his mother and the therapist.

"We'll book the surgery as early as we can, Alex needs to start speaking", I told her. I looked at my son. He hadn't seen me standing there, and seemed perfectly content to be doing what he was doing. As much as I regret my next statement, it went a long, long way into extinguishing the fire in my gut. I said plainly and matter of fact, "All the experts told me he could hear. *Every one* of them. And you know what, I *was right*. And I am not going to doubt me when it comes to him again."

That did not go over very well.

As a nurse I have seen much over the course of fourteen years. I have seen miracles, tragedy, and things that I could never explain. I have held the hands of family members as their loved one died. I have comforted wives, husbands, children and friends of the sick and dying. I remain as stoic as I can because it is my job to be there for them and emotions only make it more difficult. It is hard for me when it is my job to be the person there for them and hold back my own feelings at the same time.

I have held people who were alone as they died, and told them that it is okay to go. The precept that no one should die alone is something that one of my mentors taught me, and thirteen years later I am still appreciating just how valuable that lesson is.

People who should have left the hospital haven't, and those who should have succumbed to their disease, somehow left healthy. I have seen people code, and have saved them with CPR, compressing a stopped heart and smiling as it began to beat on its own. I made a difference. I have done all that, and still to this day it is so hard to look at my eight year son and know that as irrational as it is, my greatest failure as a nurse and health care provider sits across from me at the table *every single* day.

Shortly after his birth on August 3rd 2000, as he was whisked away by a nurse, I could tell something wasn't right. He was placed on the warming table and stayed *blue* just a little too long. An oxygen mask was being held across his face, and he was being stimulated to breathe deeply. I didn't hear his first cry for what seemed like an eternity, and I started to panic until I heard him breathe. When Alex cried, my anxiety lifted. He stayed on the table, pinked up and looked as beautiful as I had imagined.

All of my children were named while still inside their mother, and although some might call it cheating by ultrasound, I call it "I have to paint the room, what color do I need?" Each child had their name firmly in place before they ever looked outside of mommy and into the bright big lights of the delivery room into daddy's waiting hands. My children were addressed by the names chosen for them so that when they arrived on delivery day, they *knew* who they were.

Alexander's name came to me as I was sitting in the doctor's office one afternoon in early May of 2000. Debate raged back and forth as to what name to give him, and each of us had ideas that the other didn't really like. I was sitting there reading National Geographic and the feature piece was a long biographical account of the great Macedonian king and conqueror, Alexander the Great. Although ancient Greece was unified by his father, Philip II, Alexander went further on to extend the Macedon empire eastward to the periphery of what is now modern India. The name means, "protector of men", and appears in the Bible as the man who helps Jesus bear the cross on the journey to Golgotha.

Knowing all that, it fell into place, and when I presented my thoughts on the name to his mother, she agreed that it indeed was a good choice. From that day forward, the little lump (as all the children were referred to until we named them) became known as Alexander.

Alex made it out of delivery and was soon drinking as he should, and all seemed well. Later that day the first hints of jaundice were evident, and although I know in most cases it is a benign condition that clears itself over the course or a few days, this was something different.

His blood test came back with a high bilirubin, and I was alarmed. Bilirubin (or Billy Ruben for you fans of Silence of the Lambs), is a breakdown product of blood metabolism and is yellow in color. As it rises it deposits in the skin (jaundice), or is evident in the sclera or white of the eye (commonly referred to as icteric). The higher the level (and on discharge from the hospital Alex's level was fourteen), the more jaundiced and lethargic the child becomes. Alex was yellow, and somewhat slow, but otherwise was he arousable so when the doctors came in to discharge him on the fourth, I was more than apprehensive.

Being trained as a transplant RN (liver and kidney to be more precise) made me very aware of the wealth of issues a high bilirubin count would bring to a young brain. I had seen so many adults with encephalopathy, and the confusion and lethargy it brings, that I knew what would happen if the numbers rose any higher.

After a long and animated talk with three doctors and a

few nurses in the unit telling them that I thought Alex would be better served staying another day or so to make sure the number didn't go any higher. The doctor said, "It's fourteen, Mr. McGrath. He is eating and alert, just put him in the sun for a few days, the bilirubin will break down and he'll be fine. If he gets lethargic, bring him back."

He was already lethargic in my mind, but, what the fuck did I know? I told them one last time that I had a ton of experience with toxic levels and I wanted him to stay *one* more day to make sure he was processing and breaking down the deadly chemical. "He'll be fine, bring him in for blood test in a week. The levels will be normal by then. And you're only covered by insurance until today."

Insurance. Sure. Okay. You guys are the experts, not me.

So we went home, and I took the advice to heart. That day was bright and sunny, and not a single cloud was floating in the sky. The air was hot but breathable, and since we had a front and backyard at the time, it was easy to put Alex in the sunlight. He seemed okay, and for the first day my worry tapered a bit.

The next day started out much as I thought it would. Jon and Julia were busy being toddlers and doting over the now yellow-orange figure of their brother, telling him how great it was to see him. Orange. His color was wrong. My in-laws came over early and I went out to the store to pick up a few things knowing he was safe in the hands of grandma and grandpa. Besides, I needed to get out of dodge for a few minutes anyway. Three kids and one was orange! I went out thinking as soon as I get back, he's going to the MD.

An hour went by and I returned home and went to take Alex from his grandpa. Something was wrong. He was limp, not moving and sleeping way too soundly. As much as it is wrong to say this, this has been the only time my kids have been in the car and not buckled into a car seat. I didn't care if I got a ticket, arrested or both. His mother held Alex and I drove as fast I could to the hospital. He didn't move at all the whole way there. By then, it was too late. He was symptomatic and I knew what it could mean.

After getting to the hospital and being told I had to wait, the Bronx in me came pouring out. Badly, loudly and to such effect that we went *straight* into an examination room. The doctor came back and I started in on the past two days; she ordered blood and told me to wait as stat is about twenty minutes. Good, finally some action. By then, Alex was stirring as various nurses and doctors poked at him. And that in and of itself was a good thing. Twenty minutes became thirty and thirty became forty-five. The rage inside bubbled out and I made a phone call to the lab.

No one in urgent care knew that I was the evening supervisor on their transplant floor, and I didn't feel the need to tell them either. I did that simply because I was a father at that point, and a very concerned one at that. I also figured that the less people thought I knew, the more I could see if what I was getting was a consistent line of bullshit.

I called a friend in the lab, told them what was going on, and I was told that the order was urgent not stat, and it wasn't done yet. I asked him for a favor after telling him it was my newborn son's blood and I needed to know. He pushed the specimen through for me (and later that month he enjoyed a nice dinner and drinks courtesy of moi.)

I sat back and waited, and when a nurse came in to check on Alex I asked, "Any labs yet? It's been almost an hour?" I got the response I knew I would get, "No sir, not yet. I don't know what the holdup is." The doctor came in and basically said that she had no idea why the lab wasn't done but she would check. The phone in the exam room rang.

I picked it up and they looked at me as if to say, *who* the hell are you to answer the phone? I thanked Jerry and told the doctor, "Bili is 29, can you admit him *now* please?"

At that point as they were saying I had no business taking that call, I put my ID on and said that as an RN, *his* father and his nurse I most certainly did since it was *me* that fixed the fuck up on the order. (I did get reprimanded on that, but really who gave a shit, this was my child.) They found him a room and up he went to be put under the Ultraviolet lamps to start the breakdown of the toxic substance in his blood.

Three days and three nights passed. And soon his numbers were better as was his color (I have a hard time dressing him in orange even now), so we took him home and soon all was normal, I suppose.

All was well until the test results came back, and the long

road that we started Alex on began.

After years of therapy and treatments, different schools and a lot of work by everyone, Alex is where he is now. He is a delightful if not normally difficult and typical eight year old boy. He still doesn't fully look people in the eye when he speaks to them, but he hugs and kisses as he should.

He is empathetic and loving and everything a father could want. Speaking about things at times makes the emotions and the past flood into me like torrents in a tropical rain storm. When I look at him, I remember what it took to get him where he is now, and I am as uncertain of the future now as I was then. He struggles with things, but he makes his point very well known. He is loud and often brash and quite opinionated. He is so unlike his dad.

I know that one day he will be as successful a man as he is capable of and the possibilities are endless. The skills and knowledge he exhibits daily are mind-boggling to me, and anyone who ever said he was retarded and would need constant care should go back to school and learn something new. Parents often rely solely on what experts say, but isn't the reality clear to us that parents are really the experts on their children?

The song *Ghost rider* by Neil Peart is prophetic for me to hear as I drive with my kids. For all of them, shadows have indeed passed the many roads we have traveled, and life will reveal more. And you know what? That's okay. It really is. The kids have been through a lot in their short lives, and as each day begins, new challenges present themselves to all of them. Alex wakes up first each morning and starts the day as if his life is new and fresh. I think for him sunsets are left behind as each day begins anew.

So after all of this, how does it tie into the whole hero aspect I started with? It's easy, actually. I told him not too long ago that Daddy isn't a hero at all. Heroes aren't glamorous people who sell their names so money can be had. They aren't the handsome actors and actress that make movies and television shows, or the championship athlete who scores with one second left to win a game. And a hero isn't a dad who loves his kids.

Heroes, Alex, are everyday people who do extraordinary things. Heroes are pilots who land their crafts safely when crippled and save all those aboard. Heroes are teachers who use skills to teach children no one ever thought could learn. Heroes are those who sit in a lab for years to find new cures for diseases and a medicine to help eradicate the dreaded cancer that Daddy hates so much. Those are heroes for most people, Alex. But for me it is very simply stated.

To me a hero is an eight year old boy who loves his family and deals with what life tosses at him. Alex, I am not a hero. You, my son, you are mine. And one day you will read this and understand why.

I am not a hero, Alex. Daddy does his job, as he is supposed to. Grow up and be the one thing I want for you.

Be far better than me.

No, Alex, I am not a hero at all.

All I am is your daddy.

What Happens in an Instant?

What happens in an instant? Lots of things I suppose. For example, a picture is taken and instantly in this age of digital technology, a perfect reproduction appears before you. Your eye blinks, your heart beats, and you are able to pick up a fork an instant after your brain relays the message. Life also changes in an instant. You find out that you are going to be a parent, and instantly your life becomes something new. Serious illness changes your life as it makes you focus on the most primitive drive the body has: to survive no matter what.

When you see headlights in your rearview mirror an instant before maximum impact, your life changes at the very moment you hear that *crunch*...

The day after Christmas in 1998 was a typical cold and uneventful wrap of the previous day's festivities. Julia was just six months old, beautiful and smiling all the time and Jonathan was in the devilish period commonly referred to as the terrible twos. Plans had been made months before to drive to south Jersey and visit Julia's godfather and his family at their home in Toms River. I was debating between which of the two cars to take as the drive was about two hours long and I thought maybe if I took the Caddy (we had a Sedan De Ville, old but big) it might be a smoother ride. Our other car was a smaller brand new Chevy Cavalier, and since the car seats were already strapped in, I decided that it was easier to just leave well enough alone and just take it instead.

We strapped the kids into their car seats and left shortly after 9:30 a.m. The day was crisp but not unbearably cold, and once all were settled in, the drive went by without a hitch. We arrived at our destination safe and sound, and for us it was just another Christmas day as the kids got to sit under another Christmas tree and play as the adult mingled and talked. All in all, it was a very good visit.

Julia's godfather, Captain Jerry, is the father of a dear

friend of mine, and someone who when I first met him, made me feel as if he knew me his whole life. I had met his daughter some thirteen years before when I was twenty and working as a furniture installer for a computer company. Now, The Captain was seeing his goddaughter for the second time. I never quite got used to calling him by his first name (Jerry), and for years I always addressed him as Sir or Mr. D. He always laughed at that fact. He told me his friends called him Captain, so I used that moniker instead, being uncomfortable calling him anything other than that term of endearment.

When it came time to name godparents I called him on the phone and told him that I wanted him to be Julia's godfather and that I wouldn't take no for an answer. When he asked why, there were a wealth of reasons so I did my best to explain why I chose someone twenty-five years my senior.

For as long as we'd known each other, the Captain has had heart disease. Bypass surgery was never an option due to the blocked areas of his heart, and he took numerous medications to keep himself in check. I always viewed him as somewhat of a second father figure and I wanted to make sure that I did everything I could to keep him on Earth as long as possible. I was a new nurse at the time, and had been working with transplant and open heart surgery patients, and the prospect of him having another heart attack was just too much to think about.

So, being the completely rational person I am, I did the only thing I could. I named him the godfather, and told him that starting now he had this title and it was his job to make sure he danced with his goddaughter at her wedding. He agreed after laughing out loud for a bit. He was honored, and quite frankly, so was I.

We had a great visit that day, but as things would have it, it can all change in an instant. The headlights were in the rearview mirror, and immediately before the impact my first words weren't "Oh my God" or "NO!" They were "HOLY FUCK!"

Holy fuck came out of my mouth as a white Toyota slammed into us at what has now been determined as 65 miles per hour. There was a sickening sound as the rear of the car was destroyed in a flash. I can still hear the plastic and metal, each destructive sound unique in its own way. The impact jolted the kids and their mom who were strapped in, and as luck would have it my hands turned the car to the right, and at the exact moment as I corrected to keep the car straight, the other car hit us again this time on the driver's side front, and it was at that point that the airbag hit me in head and the car started to slide across four lanes of traffic.

Comfortably Numb, and it was 6:11 p.m. That was the song on the radio, and the time that stood still on the clock. To this day whenever I hear that song (which is on, in my opinion one of the top five albums of all time), I think of exactly what it is that happened on December 26th, 1998. It is very hard to listen to that track without having a wealth of memories flood into my head. Oftentimes, I simply change the station, or turn the radio off.

Sliding sideways, the kids screaming, their mother screaming louder, and I was blind. The airbag went off in a muzzle flash of sparks, air and what I can only describe as the smell of gunpowder. The impact of the bag deploying was so hard that it propelled me backward, and broke the back of my seat. Ultimately, it was the force of the airbag pinning me back and wedging the car seats between my big body and the kids that saved them from horrible injury. In effect, it cushioned the blow, so that as we hit the far guardrail and began to tumble down the hill, they were protected as if wrapped in a large roll of bubble wrap.

Have you ever heard glass explode? If you haven't, I don't recommend it. Safety glass is designed to shatter so that as it breaks, is doesn't become like a knife and slice and dice. It splinters into millions of tiny pieces, each looking somewhat like a sharp, slick diamond. Glass is glass and it cuts no matter what. At the point of first contact the rear window exploded like a bomb, and those millions of tiny fragments hit everything in sight. In the end the most serious of the cuts were from the flying shards that hit all of us. None of us escaped the wrath of the angry glass.

The guardrail gave way under the weight of the car as we slammed into it sideways. We hit it at full speed and as I heard the passenger door crumple, we were propelled up. I love rollercoasters and it took me years to get back on them after this little ride. Once I got back on the Cyclone for the first time on a visit to New York some six years later, I was hooked again. Close your eyes and imagine being in the lead car, at the top of the first precarious drop and you can see the bottom beckoning. The car went up, the guardrail acting like a springboard, and for what seemed like a minute (in reality it was probably three maybe four seconds tops), we were in the air. It seemed as if we were just floating. I knew we weren't dead because I could hear my children and their mother screaming as we were weightless before the car began an angry descent into a ravine.

There is a moment just before you realize what is about to happen that you try to make peace with yourself. *This is it* you tell yourself, you aren't getting out of it, and you hope and pray (something I still did periodically, but not as I used to) that it won't hurt much, and that your children aren't hurt or die with you. I knew that this wasn't my time to leave; I wasn't alone as I always knew I would be. My life played out before me on an open channel of memories and the only thing I remember saying to myself was, "If this is it, God, let them all be okay, please."

...*CRASH,* roll...the roof crumbled and the descent down the hill began, and *pop* the windshield was no more as the sound it made was loud and frightening. I had no idea how far we were going to go, and the only thing I heard was the car as it became a battered shell of itself. I couldn't hear the kids anymore, or their mother. I heard myself screaming, and I tasted my own blood as it ran down my face. Blood has this metallic almost coopery taste, and I wonder what the draw for vampires is. Frankly, it tastes terrible, and I don't recommend trying vampirism in the future. We were all pinned into our seats, mine was twisted and wedging the kids in and then the car turned again. The roof caved in more, and I thought this is what it feels like to be inside a trash compactor.

Here I was, talking to God. Well, talking isn't the best word to use, but I was doing something. How can we survive, God? Why are you taking my kids *now*? Why? Why? Can you tell me *why*? The answer I got was about what I expected at that time: *silence*. Silence from God, and the sound of a broken, dying engine whirring in the background as the wheels screeched loudly

We tumbled down the hill, much like clothes in a hot dryer, and with each successive flip the car became smaller and smaller as pieces either flew off or compressed inward. When we finally stopped on the last tumble the roof was collapsed around us, stopping thankfully on the top of the car seats above where the kids were. I was face down with my nose in grass, which is funny to think of now because I was turned and facing squarely into where the broken gaping maw of the driver's side window was. I could hear the engine still racing at top speed, and I remember hearing a swarm of bees. They were loud and irritating and I was stunned to think that bees would be alive in the middle of winter. The kids were screaming loudly, but I couldn't get to them. I was trapped between the now completely destroyed roof of the car, thousands of pieces of shattered safety glass and the ground on which we rested. The car was upside down.

Time seemed to stop, and for a while it did as the clock was frozen forever on 6:11. What seemed like an eternity in all actuality lasted somewhere between fifteen and thirty seconds. More than ten years after that night, I can still hear crunching and breaking glass at night as I fall sleep. That happens less and less now, but for quite some time it was constant. The bees never existed, but I can tell you that as a result of banging my head hard on the last turn of the car, my brain must have sloshed from one side to the other and knocked me completely silly. I remember the numbness in my face and head, and how slow everything moved, as if the world had given me a giant whiff of ether and the slow motion camera was in full effect. My head felt heavy and I was smelling the grass, and hearing the screams wasn't what snapped me into action.

I was strapped in, my eyes were stinging and the blood was blinding me more. I was stunned, but realized that I was still alive. I felt no pain in my neck, back or legs, but I felt as if my head weighed 100 pounds. I was lying there and began to look for an escape because I realized I could smell something in the air. I noted the sweet odor of antifreeze as it was pouring out of the radiator, and engine oil was burning against the hot metal of the now destroyed engine. I tried shaking the bees out of my head, but that was fruitless. As I started to move it was then that it fully hit me.

What I smelled was gas. A lot of it.

I tore my seat belt off and got out the only way I could, through the rear door directly behind me. I saw the shattered remains of the car for the first time. Some people on the road who witnessed the accident were staring down at me screaming and yelling at them that I wasn't dead and my family was trapped. Two young men in their twenties were already on the other side of the car removing my daughter, my then wife already resting on the ground with a hurt back.

I had torn the rest of the rear driver side door off, and had Jon firmly in my arms making sure he was alive and well. He had multiple glass injuries to his face, but the fact that he was screaming and clutching me indicated that everything was working well and that the car seats did their job.

An older couple took the kids from us and held them as I tried to calm down, which was no easy task I might add. I was able to look at what had happened, and it astounds me to this day what I saw. We had rolled almost seventy-five feet into a ravine, through a fence and came to rest five feet from a concrete drainage basin, which had we rolled into it...I think you get the picture.

I was frantic, but alive. The firefighters came and grabbed me and shoved me on a backboard, and within maybe fifteen minutes, Jon and I were headed to a local hospital. He was strapped to my chest; I found out later that Julia was with her mom, strapped to her as well. I barely felt the EMT start the large bore IV lines that tore into my veins, and I remember talking the whole ride there. I asked one of the medics if there were bees in the ambulance as I could hear them buzzing. He paid me no mind at that point.

We went straight into trauma, Jonathan was whisked away for X-rays and I went to have CAT scans of my head and neck. X-rays were taken to make sure my neck was intact, and I kept asking about everyone else. I was assured all were awake and alive, and that, all in all, we were pretty lucky. I suppose at the time I wasn't feeling that way, and now my back was hurting badly and I couldn't turn. The scans were negative, and the neck collar and straps were removed. I was given permission to stand, because quite frankly all of the fluid they gave me had filled my bladder and I had to go. There was *no way* anyone was going to catheterize me if I could help it. I was able to stand and fill the bottle and before I handed it to the nurse I remarked that at least there was no visible blood and that was good. She dipped it, and it was clear, meaning I had no lacerations to the kidney or bladder. Good, I could walk and pee.

What a good thing so far.

The kids checked out fine, and except for superficial blast injuries, both were OK. Their mom was cleared as well, and my sister was racing from Queens to come take us home. My now late uncle Jimmy, my Aunt Diane and cousin Michael all got to see me as I was still strapped down, bloody broken and quite frankly a mess. I was waiting for the CAT scan results and still had on the neck collar.

All three were supportive and anything I needed they got for me. I never forgot the fact that when I called them, (the only number I remembered was theirs, I couldn't remember my address) they came and took the kids until I was on my feet.

My sister and her friend came in a minivan, met my aunt and uncle, and once the kids were brought back to me and my ex wife, we piled into the quiet van and they drove us home. From what I remember I mumbled a lot, and was trying to get embedded glass out of my scalp. I had angry acne like holes in my face where little pieces of glass once slept. They had to be removed. One by one, piece by piece. A little over a year later I was still finding small pieces under my scalp, a constant reminder of what was probably the most frightening night I ever had.

After we were dropped off and the kids finally settled into bed, I lay in the dark trying to sleep but not having too much luck. The both of us lay there, my wife was sound asleep and practically motionless, and I looked at the closed door of my closet and I could smell the fear coming off of me.

When you lay in the dark after an experience in which your life not only flashes before you, but you actually bargain with whoever God really is, your mind wanders. I had this incessant buzzing and heavy headed feeling, and no matter how I turned or tried to position myself to get comfortable, sleep wouldn't come.

I wanted to sleep so badly, and as I lay on my back and watched the ceiling in the dead of night, it was then that I saw the black phantom that lurks in the shadows. He tried to be inconspicuous, but I saw him. And when he was aware that I knew, he grew in stature and stared straight at me.

I thought I saw the first glimpse by the door of the closet, and I saw the shadow on the ceiling grow. All I could see was a black hooded shape, and a twisted, hideous smile. I cringed, but my eyes couldn't close. He *wanted* me to see, to be aware that this time he had missed. And as I looked and saw the awful grin break through the darkness, I started to speak to him.

"You have no business here, leave." I spoke in barely a whisper, and as I did the smile got wider. I spoke louder and more firmly, and finally when he wouldn't leave I started screaming out loud. My wife woke up and looked at me with half closed eyes as I screamed in anger at the ceiling.

She asked who was I screaming at and I pointed at the ceiling.

"Look, *he's right there, I see him, and he missed! Get the hell out of my house, now!*" I could tell she was scared because she kept saying over and over that she didn't see anything, and I told her that I did.

I was out of control, screaming in rage and fear and wondering what would happen now if I did fall asleep. As I started to get up and out of the bed the shadow just faded into the ceiling and disappeared.

I never figured out if I was hallucinating from hitting my head, or if he was actually there. I can tell you that he does exist though. He lurks and skulks about, and every now and again I still see him.

The aftermath of the accident was an endless stream of insurance companies and doctors. I went to see a therapist to help through the post traumatic stress, and even today I often jump when I see a white car behind me, or coming on my left. The kids have no recollection of the event.

I don't like anything that happens in an instant anymore. Not instant drinks, foods, or answers to questions.

Sometimes, waiting isn't so bad tireless reader.

Think of what can happen.....in an instant.

For Mischa...

I was once asked to write something happy that was filled with butterflies and puppies. Although I would like to write only the highest of highs all the time instead of the lowest of lows, sometimes the only thing that you can put down on paper is as difficult to write as is it is to read.

I was an assistant nurse manager on a surgery wing at a major hospital on Long Island. I had been a transplant nurse for just over two years when the commute to the city became too much on me physically, so I chose to change jobs. Starting out as a night shift floor RN, it quickly became apparent to me that there was a lack of strong leadership on the middle shift. Being the Type-A personality that I am, I simply asked my manager what I needed to do to step up the next level. The answer was a non-descript, "Apply and go through the process". Soon thereafter I applied, went on a spate of interviews with the evening staff and upon their recommendation (and much to the delight of the big boss herself), I was moved into the management spot. From soup to nuts, it took two months.

At times, running a shift can be easy. Most times it isn't and one has to counterbalance the needs of the many over the needs of the one. Staffing is always an issue, and I quickly learned who worked best with whom, how to pair the staff together to be productive and not get in each other's way. Most nurses are territorial, and their patient is *their* patient, and pairing two strong willed individuals doesn't work. Some staff moved to other floors, others were hired, and soon enough we had a good group who worked together for the common good.

I was sitting in the office one evening, which was a rare occurrence as on most days I had a patient load of ten or twelve people. I liked to be hands-on with all the transplants. I was planning the schedule when a doctor knocked and asked me if I was really a hockey fan. Smiling and pointing to my black leather Ranger jacket my answer was, "Yes, I am, and I still skate one or two nights a week." He introduced himself in a heavy Russian accent, "I'm Dr. Ostrovsky, and I am new here". He held out his hand which I shook firmly. I said to him, "Nice to meet you." At that point he told me his friends called him Michael, (although his name on the hospital ID said Mikhail) and he said he would like to talk to me later. "Sure", I said. "It's not like either of us is leaving anytime soon."

With that he left to see his group of patients and I put my head back down and got back to work. A simple interchange between us led to the birth of a friendship.

Michael was a new resident on the transplant service and was busy introducing himself to other staff. I left the office and made rounds in each room as I would normally do on the days when I didn't have an assignment. After seeing all the patients and staff, I was satisfied that the evening would go along smoothly, I walked over to Michael and asked him who his favorite team was. He laughed and said "The Devils" in his heavy accent. "I'm a big Ranger fan, but I love the game, so I won't hold it against you," I said.

He was reviewing charts and once he was done, he started asking me the usual battery of questions that people getting acquainted usually do. "Are you from New York? Where do you skate? How long have you been here?" and so on. I answered most of his questions, and he began to tell me that he was a new resident at the hospital and didn't know many of the nurses. He had found the right person to talk to and as I showed him around the unit, I introduced him to my staff, and anyone else that was there.

What I quickly learned was that Michael was in the midst of having to repeat all of his medical training over again. Once a Gynecological surgeon in Russia, he was forced to do a residency again here in the states. He wound up on our unit as part of the revolving door of residents, and having a skilled surgeon (although he wasn't doing operating yet) on the floor was a bit of a comfort to me. I learned soon enough to trust him as a doctor, and he learned to trust my instincts as a nurse. Once I trusted his judgment, it became much easier to work on the floor knowing that I had him around. He always gave direct answers, which is how I prefer things, and in all the time we worked together, there was never an issue between us.

Michael had a love of all sports, but particularly hockey. Once as I was sitting in the office he asked if I collected baseball cards. Quickly telling him "No, why?" he simply answered that he was an avid collector and wanted to know if I would be interested in buying and selling cards with him as a hobby. We both had young sons, and since we shared an avid love of hockey, I said, "Sure, why not?"

Once that little seed was planted, the tree blossomed incredibly fast. The ironic thing about the two of us was we were completely polar opposites on so many levels. He was short in stature standing around five feet six at best to my six foot one. He was an orthodox Russian Jew to my Irish Roman Catholic. He followed a rather strict conventional kosher diet, and well, I didn't follow any.

We shared commonalities in our love for a game, a hobby and our families. Soon Michael and his family (wife Nelly and two children, Alan and Danielle) began to spend time with my family at my home in Ronkonkoma that first summer. I had a large backyard. It was able to hold us all and let the kids run freely while we sat as adults and did what we normally did: the wives spoke and watched the kids play, and he and I would sit at the table and break open a fresh case of cards and sort out everything. Six or seven hours later we'd be done and each took his share to keep. Those summer days were easy and carefree and Michael told me a few short months after our initial meeting that if he had a brother, I would be like him.

That was a nice thing to say, and since I didn't *know* I had any brothers at that time, I viewed him as one too.

As fall came that year, Michael would come over to my house on the evenings he was on call (I lived three minutes from where we worked, and now that he is gone it doesn't really matter who knows) and we sat and watched games on the satellite dish. I had set aside a drawer in the kitchen for his food as he kept kosher and it was easier to keep things separate. I remember one night he was in the kitchen looking at everything I had and I asked what he was reading. He showed me a small symbol that indicated it was kosher and he was able to eat it, so after that first exchange it became quite easy to identify things for him.

Two and half years after he left, and some eleven years after we met, I still remember where to look for it, and what it means.

One of the things that I remember best is his voice when

he got excited. He would scream in a high squeal and curse in Russian when the Devils weren't doing well. I still think that my Alex remembers those episodes because when he gets mad he often does the same thing. I secretly think that if we went to Russia, Alex would understand the language fully.

Michael's parents finally left Russia and immigrated to Long Beach, New York where I met them as well. He had met both of my parents and extended family so it seemed logical that when they came here we would meet, as well. To this day when I look at his father and catch his eyes, I can see the pain he still carries.

There is such a wealth to tell that I really don't know what to say and what to leave out, so for the sake of space I will say we spent many days together as friends and colleagues. When I had my accident in 1998, I was still recovering from the injuries when I returned to work a week after the roll-over. I didn't realize I was limping or wincing in pain when I moved and he was the one that told me I wasn't right, that I needed to see a neurologist. Michael showed up with a basket of food for us when I couldn't get out to the store those first few days after the accident. When I needed something he was always there for me and my family.

He was there giving advice as a doctor when the little boys were born, and he was the one who tried his hardest to keep me and the family in New York when I wasn't able to make ends meet. Try as he might, I left. I left a brother, a colleague, but most of all, someone I loved as a very dear and close friend. When I left September 28, 2001, I called him and told him I would see him soon and call him a few times a week.

That is exactly what I did.

We spoke three to four times a week, sometimes briefly, sometimes for an hour or so. Things were better for my family in Florida at the time, but it certainly didn't diminish the fact that I missed my family and friends back in New York. The phone served the purpose it was invented for, and although we weren't getting together physically anymore, we were able to stay as close as two friends can be separated by 1250 miles.

In April of 2003 he called to ask if I could meet him in Tampa and spend a few days there while he attended a conference. Once I was able to get the days off, I made plans to drive to Tampa and spend a four day weekend there with him. We made plans to go see the Yankees and Rays play, have dinner and walk around the downtown area. It was on the first day I was there that I was able to see that something wasn't quite right.

More than anything he looked tired. Not a good tired but haggard and a lot slower than his normal, jovial self. We were set to go out to eat and he was muttering in Russian and looking about frantically.

"Michael," I asked him. "What the hell are you looking for?"

"Keys to car. I can't remember where they are."

Normally such things don't really bother me much. This time a small bell went off inside of me as the keys were on the television staring back at both of us. I picked them up and tossed them to him, and we made no mention of it again. We headed out to eat and then were slated to see the Yanks and Rays that night and would be meeting two other doctors for the ride. I drove all of us in my car, and since I drove the other three passengers picked up the price on the tickets.

All in all, not a bad deal!

The rest of that night I kept a careful eye on Michael and although I couldn't pick up what the problem was, I knew he wasn't the same.

"Michael, what's wrong with you, you don't look right." He answered, "I'm working and getting ready to take the medical boards. I am just tired".

I left it as it was, and made no mention of it again. After all, he was young and strong and ready to be what he wanted to be: a doctor in the United States.

We said our goodbyes and he flew home to New York, and I drove east toward my home in Viera. The whole way home I was trying to think…wonder…reason…what was the problem? I couldn't figure it out, and I never thought of the most obvious until five months later when his mother called.

I got home and my then wife asked me how Michael was. I told her I wasn't sure but that something wasn't adding up. I made mention of his forgetfulness and fatigue and she waved it off much like he did telling me I was overanalyzing things as I always did.

We spoke less and less that summer as he was hunkered down in his home cramming for the boards and I was busy working two night jobs to support the family. One day in early September of 2003, after not being able to get a hold of him and not getting any return calls from him, his mother called and left a message for me to call Michael's wife right away. I never spoke to his mother much, so for her to call me it had to be important. A wealth of visions went through my head and I was worried. I called his mother, and in broken English she said:

"Michael in hospital, call Nelly."

So I picked up the phone to call his wife, I took a pen and paper and wrote down a few words, neatly folded it, and handed to my now ex and told her to wait until I was done. She was sitting outside smoking and talking to her friend Colleen. I sat out there and dialed the phone as she looked at me and the paper folded in her palm. The two of them went on with their conversation and Nelly picked up.

I asked what happened and how bad it was. She told me he had brain surgery the previous day and wanted to tell me himself. By then I was already sitting with my head in my hands. He took the phone and in a barely audible voice I heard the words that I had dreaded, and knew were coming.

Brain tumor.

A *Gliobastoma* is the most common of the brain tumors accounting for over fifty percent of all those diagnosed. Symptoms include fainting spells (syncope) and balance and coordination difficulties, but usually the most common symptoms are progressive memory loss and personality changes.

Treatments involve using radiation surgery and chemotherapy, all of which are known simply as palliative measures, meaning that they do not provide a cure but are based on symptom control and comfort. Even if completely removed surgically and combined with the best available treatment, the survival rate for *Gliobastoma* remains very low.

Although common symptoms include seizures, headaches, nausea and vomiting and one sided paralysis, the single most prevalent symptom is a progressive memory, personality, or neurological deficiency due to frontal and/or temporal lobe involvement. Symptoms are based on where the tumor lies and most of these tumors produce no such symptoms until it has grown very large and by that time, it is too late.

The surgery, called a craniotomy, was performed the day before, and I was talking to him only a few hours after he had most of the primary tumor removed. Underneath the primary tumor was a second one, in effect like some sort of sick version of the famous matryoshka doll's everyone sees at least once in their lives.

He was weak, and asked me to speak to Nelly for further information, and as fast as one can say their name, he handed the phone to his wife. She told me that a few days before he had been at work and had gotten extremely dizzy. His boss suggested a CAT scan just to make sure he wasn't having any stroke symptoms, so he agreed and got into the machine. A few minutes later a group of doctors were hovering over him and staring at the screen. The tumor was large, and it had caused his dizziness. He was admitted and given steroids to decrease the pressure in his brain. Surgery was a scant few days later, and now I was getting the grim news.

I hung up the phone, sat on my porch and buried my face into my hands. And not soon after that as my wife and her friend sat there smoking and looking at me, I cried. For a long time they let me sit there without so much as saying a word.

Michael made it home with an action plan already in place a few days later. He was going to Duke University for experimental treatment. As a surgeon, he knew what his prognosis was, and when all calmed down and I was able to speak to him, he relayed that the one thing he wanted was to see his son make his Bar Mitzvah. He told me he would do all he could to make it until the spring of 2006.

Treatments came and went and Michael was as stable as he could be. For quite a while he had what is termed as *stable disease*. It neither grew nor shrunk and he was able to function as a doctor, but not as a surgeon. He passed his medical boards in early 2005 and was beginning to function as a successful practitioner. Treatments had continued to keep the tumor at bay, and we spoke as often as we could. I always remember listening intently as I could for any hint of change.

Tumors such as the one he had are as invasive and destructive as an advancing superior army. Not long after he passed the boards the erosive nature of the tumor had advanced to the point that one morning he woke up and couldn't move the right side of his body. His speech was slurred and he could no longer walk. The re-scan of his brain had shown that the tumor was indeed back, and even with further treatment the destruction would not stop. The doctors essentially told Michael that nothing more could be done.

I spoke to him on that day in September and he told me that he was going to make it until the Bar Mitzvah, and would I come when he asked. My answer was, "Of course I will". After all, it was the only thing I felt that I could do. His wife took the phone and stated very clearly to me what was happening. All the plans for the spring were being changed and that the new date was December 11, 2005. She asked me to come, and I agreed. That phone call was in early October.

I made plans to fly into New York on December 10th, and stay for a short time. I had to come and leave to get back to the kids. Things at home weren't good, and the longer I stayed away the worse I knew it would become. Michael went into the hospital a few short days before I arrived and he would not be making it to the ceremony. He was in the hospital with his father keeping a constant vigil. The last time I had spoken to him, Michael said something to me and I knew I had to leave as fast as I could.

He said in his broken English, slurred by understandable, "Markie, you come now, come see me now".

I hopped on the plane and rushed back to New York, not fully knowing what to expect.

The big bird touched down on December 10, 2005 on a cold, winter day. Outside it was snowing, the streets were icing, and the constant reminder of Christmas was overwhelming. I landed shortly after 9:30 am and as soon as I met my sister at the gate I was taking in everything I could. The air was crisp and sharp and the wind bit into me much as I remembered it did all those winters ago when I skated outdoors on the lake. She dropped me off for a quick hello with my mom, and I took her car and started the drive to Long Beach to meet up with Nelly and the kids. She had something she wanted me to see first before we left for the hospital.

When it became apparent to me that Michael's condition

was as bad as it was, on a rainy day in Florida I sat at my laptop and wrote a letter to the New Jersey Devils. Since he was a rabid fan and attended many functions when the team was present, I thought that maybe I could get them to sent him something. A month or so after I wrote the letter I received an email from Lou Lamariello's secretary (he is the General Manager of the Devils) stating that they had received my letter and that they needed Michael's address. I profusely thanked her and alerted Nelly. The NHL offices in New York contacted me a few months before I last saw him to find out if what I said was indeed true. When my story was verified, the NHL contacted the three area teams, and each team sent him something.

A month or so before the end came, I received a call from Michael's wife and she held the phone next to him. He was as excited as he could be and wanted to thank me. I had no idea what he was referring to. Over the course of a few months each of the teams sent him gifts via mail, and those I were aware of. This last thing that came arrived in a nondescript envelope with the New Jersey Devils address and header, and inside of it was the one thing he had always wanted.

Inside, sent by Mr. Martin Brodeur himself, was a signed, game-used jersey used by the Devils goalie in a game earlier the previous season. Michael had many pieces of memorabilia, but this was the one thing he lacked. Michael had life in his voice and he was thanking *me* for what I had done. Really, the person who did something was Martin, not me. A few months before all I did was send an email to the Devils and I did send a letter of thanks to the Devils and Martin shortly after Michael died.

I arrived at the hospital shortly after 4 p.m., Grigori, Michael's father was there waiting for me. Workmen were busy setting up a cable feed for the festivities, and Nelly was nice enough to send out for large dinners for all of us. I quickly shook Grigori's hand and entered the room. I asked to be alone with Michael for a few minutes.

In the bed was Michael, sick, dying and to say I was upset and dismayed at what I saw wouldn't do justice to the feelings inside. The steroids had bloated him almost beyond recognition and his head was twice its normal size with fluid buildup. He was lying there, moaning and I can only imagine how horrible he felt and what was going through his mind. My instinct to make the pain go away took over, but since I wasn't a nurse in that facility there wasn't much more I could do other than ring the bell and speak nurse to nurse.

I went over and took his hand, and spoke into his left ear softly. I told him I had come as I promised and without opening his eyes he said, "Thank you for coming, sit". I sat there holding the swollen hand of my friend and feeling helpless for maybe the first time as an RN. I had never had this empty feeling as a nurse before and it was overwhelming. My friend was lying there, and I couldn't help him.

There are two rules that help me deal with things as a nurse, and sometimes when I teach new nurses or try to mentor people (imagine that, *me* a mentor! I laugh at that sometimes) as they begin their careers, I state them once for effect. They are simple rules really, but they do help set parameters for me:

1). You are a nurse. In your career, you will care for many patients. Most will get better, but some of them will get sicker and die.

2). No matter what you know, how hard you work, or how skilled you are, rule #1 never changes.

On that particular day, both rules applied...and they both sucked.

I sat there for a half hour just speaking to him in as soft a voice as I could. His father had come into the room and sat in a chair and listened as I told him how well things were for me and the kids in Florida (a lie, but he didn't need to know that), and that everything would be okay. I told him I was staying there with him through the ceremony, that I had come as he asked because I loved him, and that I was there to do what whatever he wanted. He was moaning in pain; I could see how bad it was in his eyes. His nurse came in and I asked to speak to her outside.

I explained to her that I was a dear friend to Michael and a nurse as well. I asked her what the parameters on his pain control were and she gave me the typical time limit I expected to hear. I asked if it were possible to call the doctor to see if they could institute a steady low dose morphine drip for comfort as the three hour limit didn't seem like it was helping. She said she would call, and with that she gave a dose of Morphine to him. He calmly slipped into sleep.

Over the next hour Michael's mentor and sponsor arrived and we sat together and talked for the first time. We sat there and as Michael slept the rest of us had a quiet catered dinner courtesy of Nelly and the kids. The nurse arrived with a small pump and a medicated bag filled with morphine and I quietly nodded and mouthed *thank you* to her. She smiled and hung the drip then left the room. I explained to Michael's father and Dr. Petrokovsky what I had requested from the nurse. We sat there and although I know we all thought the same thing, neither of the three of us said so much as a word.

We watched the screen as his son's party was beamed in via closed circuit television. Although I know he knew we were there, and he could hear everything, he lay there and didn't move or moan. At the very least, I knew deep down that he was comfortable, and as his friend, and more importantly as a nurse, that his pain was better controlled. One of the hardest things to do is watch uncontrolled pain. In this case, since I was so close to the person experiencing it, watching it was that much harder.

The last hour I was there I sat on the bed and held his hand and didn't say much. I knew that this was the last time, at least here on this planet, that I would see him. He wasn't the same vibrant man I had come to view as a brother over the years. The cancer had already taken most of him. What was left was a mere shell of the person he had been. Slowly his abilities had been taken away, and now he was laying there in the end phase as the tumor sucked away whatever life he had left. I was sitting there watching, and hating. Not hating him, but hating the disease that was robbing him of life at thirty-seven. Watching and feeling helpless and knowing that whatever I could do wouldn't be enough.

The last thing I did before I left was walk around to the other side of bed and look at him quietly breathing and not moving. I kissed the top of his head and whispered in his ear, "Mischa...It's okay. Your family will be ok. You can leave now. I love you my friend, goodbye."

I looked at him one last time, and as the tears rolled silently down my cheeks and I stifled myself, I saw a tear roll down his face as well. And with that, I turned and left. It was the last time I saw him.

Michael died from his brain tumor on December 16th,

2005. The call came at 9 a.m. as I was driving home from work. His wife simply said that his parents and family were there and she said one of the last things he said was, "Tell Markie thank you." He slipped back into sleep, and left quietly and peacefully.

I went home and sat on the bed for a few minutes looking at some old photos of us when he was alive. I didn't need to be thanked, or feel anything other than a tremendous loss over what cancer had robbed. My tears came freely and quietly, and I sat there alone.

Now, a few years later I still think of him when the Devils play the Rangers. I see his wife and kids as often as I can and they are doing well. Pictures on the wall remind us all of who he was and what he meant to his family and friends.

Pictures don't tell one thing, though. There is a hole in all of our hearts where he used to be. I remember him as a colleague, and more importantly, as one of the best friends I ever had. And so I wrote this as much for him as I did for myself and anyone who reads it.

I miss you terribly, Michael.

Executive Decisions and Puppies

One day the kids and I were walking through the Merritt Island Mall (for those of you not familiar, it is a mall in Merritt Island, Florida) shopping for sneakers and heading for the food court. Valentine's Day was just around the corner, and since the kids knew that the Valentine's Fairy brought them chocolate hearts and small gifts, they were busy looking at a variety of candy and neatly packaged goodies. Shoes in hand, (and, if you have never been shoe shopping with four screaming kids, I suggest you try it, as it really is mind numbing) we headed toward the kids favorite place to eat for a not so hearty lunch of commercially made pizza.

After eating, we had time before we needed to get home, so we walked toward the back end of the mall where, coincidentally enough, the pet store was. Now personally, I hate them. I see small animals and birds in cages and it makes me realize how I would feel cooped up inside one of those. But, the kids like to look at the bunnies and birds, and all of the baby animals and fish, so it seemed like a relatively safe idea. I don't like looking at puppies and always do my best to walk away from the sad, forlorn faces I see staring back at me.

This day was different though. The kids were looking at the smaller breeds and asking for Daddy to bring home a Chihuahua, Maltese, and a Poodle. As I made the typical sarcastic comment I always seem to have at the tip of my tongue, "Guys, look. If I want a dog, it will be a big manly dog, not something that is smaller than my foot." I saw the saddest pair of eyes I had seen in quite a long time. There she was. She just stared and looked and didn't move much other than to track me as I watched the kids. She was a small Irish setter, and she was the cutest puppy in the store. Like an addict looking for a fix, I looked back.

The hook, as they say, had been set.

The debate inside me raged as to what to do. I didn't

want a puppy. The kids did, and if I brought one home who knew what the reaction would be. We had three cats, and I had to consider what getting a puppy would add to what already was a chaotic house. I had a double stroller with the little boys, and Jon and Julia were walking with me; as I said, "Let's go kids", I looked one more time. She lay there sad and dew-eyed much like Puss N Boots in *Shrek* as if saying, "Please *mister*. Take me home!" I stopped at the counter, asked how much she cost and had them remove her from the cage. I don't know who was more excited, the kids or the puppy.

The pet store had a small corralled area for us to sit and let my kids and the puppy interact with each other. She became full of life, and was a ball of mahogany fur as she jumped and ran around. The inner voices inside me debated as they normally do. When she tried to jump on my lap, the final nail in the *BUY ME* coffin had been driven in. Once those first few licks were started I carried her over to the sales person and said, "Okay, I lose."

Seven hundred bucks later I had a new baby to take home.

It didn't take long for the proverbial cat in the bag (or in this case a puppy in a box) to be let out as Jon and Julia tore through the door and began screaming at their mom, "*We got a puppy!*" I got the look I knew I would get, *what did you do,* along with the rolling eyes, but she said nothing. I let the puppy out of the box and as soon as I did, the cats took off as she made a beeline for them. I had brought home a mini buzz saw and life, as they say, was not quite the same. She didn't have a name yet, and that was the first thing we needed to do so that she *knew* who she was.

Each of the kids came up with names but most of them were just plain silly. Their mom and I couldn't agree on what *we* liked, and then a thought came to me. As I watched the puppy run around, I realized something. She ran around at a frenetic pace, crashing into things, chasing the kids and cats around the house, part ADD and part Schizophrenia. Then the name popped into my head. "Hey guys...what is the name of that fish you like in *Nemo*, the one that keeps bumping into things and talking all the time?"

"Dory?" the kids all said in unison.

"Exactly. Kids, this is Dory. That is what we will name

her. It's perfect."

And, for a little while, it was.

When I was a nine year old boy, my parents took my sister and me out one night to a small house in Queens. I remember that it was cold and dark outside because it was the middle of February and back then it was plain brutal and nasty in the winter. When we got to the house, much to our surprise, we were greeted by two huge Irish Setters and I could hear puppies yelping in the background. Mom and dad had brought us to one of his co-workers homes to pick out a puppy. Later that night we left with not one or two, but three! One was for my grandmother in the city, one for my other grandmother in New Jersey, and one for us.

We picked the only male that was left, the smallest of the bunch, and later when we got home, he slept in a box. We picked the name *Shannon* for him because an Irish dog deserved an Irish name. Besides, he was a good dog and the name just kind of fit.

We had Shannon all through my grammar and high school days, and everyone on the block knew who he was. He was small for a setter, but had a great demeanor and temperament. He was quiet and for some strange reason in the summers he liked sleeping out on the fire escape. I grew up with him and on most nights he either slept on the floor in my room or on the bed with either my mom or me.

When I was nineteen I came home one day from the rink to a very sad mom and a very sick dog. I rushed him over to the vet. After a day of exams and scans we were told that the cancer inside of him was overwhelming and the best option was to euthanize him. My mom was heartbroken, as was Dad, and neither could go to the vet that day to say goodbye. So, I took Kelly in the tape mobile (my first car was an Olds Delta 88, and a few of my readers remember the duct tape around the roof) and we drove over to 234th Street to the vet's office.

He was in a cage, sick and very sad looking. I remember looking at his now white muzzle and thought, *When did you get so old?* He could barely lift his head, but when he saw Kelly and me he tried to stand. We were both crying and I think inside he was too. He licked our faces one last time, and I said *Goodbye*. He knew what was going to happen, and somehow the look in his eyes told me that it was ok. He was in a lot of pain and none of us wanted to see him linger any longer. Kelly and I ran out of the vet crying uncontrollably.

When we got home my mother said that as soon as we left the vet called my mom to see if Kelly and I were both okay because of how upset we were when we left the office. He told her that he made sure Shannon was comfortable, and after a short injection, Shannon left us.

Almost twenty-five years later I remember the day he died. May 15, 1984. At that point, it was the hardest day I had ever experienced.

Sometimes as a parent I exercise what I call an executive decision. My dad never used the term but often he made decisions that were his and his alone. For no other reason than that, he decided to do something, and he did.

A short week or so after Shannon left I came home from work and my dad was sitting on the stoop (for those not familiar with the term, the stoop is the stairs in front of a building or house) and he had a *new* dog. He was still a puppy, but much bigger than Shannon. He was already 65 pounds, deep mahogany and long flowing rich hair. Dad had taken it upon himself to replace our loss with a new dog. He had driven upstate and picked up this dog earlier in the day, and sat there waiting for us to come home so he could surprise us.

Surprise indeed. I had just gotten used to *not* having a dog anymore and was still sad over Shannon dying. This dog jumped up and almost knocked me completely over. Mom wasn't prepared either, but I think that my dad was so despondent over Shannon he did what he thought was best to ease his pain.

So, a few short days later we had a new dog, a big purebred setter this time. We decided again to give the dog a Celtic name, and since he was so deeply red we settled on Rory. Rory means red, and he really was. I thought Clifford might work, but someone else had named their big red dog Clifford and wrote a series of books on him. I didn't think copyright infringement was a good idea.

Rory grew quickly into a majestic specimen. Tall and proud, deeply red and with a flowing coat, he pranced around like he was the best. I remember watching films of the great racehorse Secretariat and how one could see the confidence and presence the great champion had. In some animals, self awareness and confidence is seen, and in my dog it just oozed out of him. He was big by setter standards, but he was such a gorgeous animal. He had his quirks though. Often in the morning I would find him walking in a circle or staring blankly into space. Sometimes he was friendly with other dogs, and other times he would completely lose control. We never could figure out *why* he was as he was, until the seizures started one day when he was four.

I remember watching helplessly as he seized, and the vets answer was medication. We tried it for a while but the dose was so big that when we took mom to the vet to get him, he didn't recognize us. We told the vet that we couldn't have him live like that and the vet did something totally unexpected.

He took Rory to his farm in upstate New York and adjusted his meds. He didn't charge us a dime. When we got the dog back six weeks later he was fine and his old self. The vet did tell us that should he have clusters of seizures again, he would probably die from them, but that the medicine was working well and the goal now was to wean him off to a very small dose.

For six months Rory was himself and all was good. One Friday night a few friends and I went to Lido Beach to a club called California. We were there until four a.m., and since I was the designated driver we all got home safe and sound shortly after five a.m.

When I walked in the door my mother was awake and the dog didn't rush to the door as he normally did. I knew what it meant, and when I asked what had happened my mom simply said, "He had a big seizure and we took him to the emergency center. He died in the car." She turned and went into her room and closed the door.

I went into mine and much to my surprise no tears flowed. I tried, but they didn't come. I think deep down I knew that it would happen and I had mourned him six months before when the vet took him in. The next Monday morning I called the vet as I usually did to give him the weekly update. I simply said, "Rory had a massive seizure on Friday and died in the car as my sister drove him into Manhattan. My mom was with him. Thank you for everything."

The silence on the other end of the phone was deafening to me. The doctor said, "Thank you for telling me. I'm sorry."

And with that he hung up the phone.

A week later a nice hand written letter arrived to my mom from the doctor. He really tried his best it said. He thanked us for allowing him to care for the dog, and he was glad that for six months Rory had his family.

When I read that letter, that's when the tears flowed. It was also when I decided I didn't want another dog.

Now, here I was a father myself using executive decision to buy my kids the one thing I said I never wanted again...a dog. The kids were happy though, and although I knew that somehow my decision of one would come back to bite me in my ample ass, I simply decided that maybe it would work out and the dog would be a good fit.

Dory was clumsy and got into everything. I took her to a puppy school and she graduated with a degree in higher training. She learned to sit, stay and walk safely without a leash. But the leash laws in Florida were pretty strict so walking her without one wasn't an option. Puppies are funny creatures. At first they are cute little furry things that follow you around and pee all over the place. Soon they become housebroken, scratching at the door or grabbing the leash as if to say... "Take me to the can *now* or I'll shit on your floor."

But mostly what they do is grow.

And Dory grew. The bigger she got, the more she rough housed with the kids. She got too rough at times, and when I brought that to the vet's attention she told me that Dory viewed the kids as other puppies and she was playing as if they were part of her litter. Fair enough I thought. The problem was, she was grabbing the kids around the neck with her mouth and at times she dragged Aidan across the floor. It became quite evident eight months into the great puppy experiment that something had to give.

The kids were afraid of her, and she was spending way too much time in her kennel. I worked nights and the kids didn't want to play with her anymore, she was simply much too rough with them.

So, after debating the pros and cons of having her, I did the only thing I could do. I made an executive decision again. I told the kid's mom that I had found a place called Brevard Setter rescue, and that I thought we should give Dory to a family that could give her what we couldn't. I had made the call earlier in the day and they agreed to come and get her and all her supplies.

I went to work that evening at three p.m. The Setter Rescue came promptly at 6:30 p.m. When I got home, she was gone. The kennel, her leash, all her toys and Dory were gone; no signs of her were left.

The kids woke up the next morning and for the first time in many months it was a quiet morning. The great puppy experiment had ended.

Executive decisions made by Daddy don't always work for the best. My new rule is no new pets. Unless it's a blue Beta in a fish bowl named Max. That is something I can probably handle.

Great Grandma, Revenge and Spooks

One of my favorite all time movies is the 1939 Classic *The Wizard of Oz*. Every year since I was a small boy, I would go and see it come to life on the large screen, or I would watch it on the television. Usually it played around Thanksgiving, just before the long march through all of the animated Christmas specials came on. I never quite knew why I liked it so much. (Although now as an adult I can say that it must have been the way Judy Garland sang. All these years later, she still totally blows me away.) But I did and still do. I have seen it numerous times with my kids, and each one has a favorite character.

There is a scene in which the Cowardly Lion, scared out his wits yet again, closes his eyes and repeats the line... "I do believe in spooks, I do believe in spooks, I do, I do, I do..." I can tell you that my hairy, petrified friend is indeed right. There are such things as ghosts, spooks or spirits, and the following is my offer of proof to you my faithful reader.

I come from a small sometimes eccentric family in New York City. I remember long since dead aunts and uncles and lost cousins from my early years. As children my sister and I went into Manhattan every Sunday to grandma's house to see my mother's parents when they lived in the projects behind Lincoln Center. They had a small apartment on the tenth floor, and on the sixth floor lived my great grandmother, Katherine.

Great grandma was a small woman but someone full of life. She seemed to enjoy the weekly visits her great grandchildren had with her. Many days were spent sitting at her table drinking milk and eating Social Tea biscuits after dinner. An old black and white television set sat on a small table in her living room, and I can still picture the ancient porcelain doll that sat neatly dressed and proper looking on her always made bed. As I look back at the long gone days of my youth I realize...I miss her, as I do all of those who have died and touched my life somehow.

I never really knew much about her as a person until very recently, but I do remember her and some of the things she did that made life a bit interesting. My aunt DeeDee (you know it sounds strange but I can't call her anything other than that. Diane is her name, but since I was small DeeDee it has been and shall remain) is the historian in the family. When I thought of putting this to paper she was the person I contacted for a little fact checking. So, thanks to an email and a very gracious aunt, I can relate a bit about grandma before I get to the days surrounding her death and a bit of revenge on her part.

Katherine was born in New York City in 1898, and as most people from her era, she was a survivor. She survived the death of two husbands, World Wars, the Great Depression and the streets of the city. She was a small woman, and by the time I was sixteen I had almost a foot in height over her. By all accounts she was the one that my mother, aunts and family depended on for a good lunch (she didn't believe in my staple of peanut butter and jelly), and baked a variety of cookies and cakes for her family so dessert was always readily available. I remember many days eating at her table where I was never disappointed. I consider myself lucky to have had her as part of my life for sixteen years.

The rule was don't tangle with great grandma, and that rule is now carried on by my mother; the kids know not piss off Nana. She believes in revenge and getting even, but she had such a subtle way of doing it. She held grudges quietly, often for years, and I often think to myself that *maybe* I hold them sometimes because it is a genetic trait passed on by her.

All these years later, I can still remember the smell of her pot roast or turkey, and I fondly think of the days I spent with family on Amsterdam Avenue in New York. I have gone there many times since then. The old building is much the same as it was some thirty years after I last walked through it.

Toward the end of her life, great grandma lived with my grandmother (mom's mother) and my grandfather on the thirteenth floor of a high rise co-op in the Bronx. Nothing about how we met as a family changed much and in fact it made it easier to see everyone on the weekends. I was getting older and didn't really like to go there all the time, but I can see now that it was an important part of my life and who I am now as a father. I wouldn't trade any memories of any of my grandparents for a bank full of money or fame.

I think back and remember calling the house, and when great grandma answered, she didn't remember who I was. I would say to my mother afterwards that grandma doesn't know who I am anymore. It was sad to think then at sixteen years old, that my grandma could just lose all recollection of things. I understand now at forty-four, and being a nurse for fifteen odd years (some years are indeed odd, some things I have seen as a nurse are stranger still), that in some cases the mind does go. Dementia, Alzheimer's, Stroke and high blood pressure lead to memory problems and I cannot say for sure which she had. I do know that she was full of life up until the very end, but I'm sure that she remembered all of us in her own way on the day she passed away.

As she advanced into her ninetieth year, Katherine began to fade. She had lived ninety long years without having a major surgery or illness of any kind. I find that to be quite remarkable. Two weeks or so before the end, she began calling my great aunt Jessie in Arizona telling her that she was dying and she needed to come to New York to say goodbye. From all accounts, Aunt Jessie was a tightwad. She refused her crying mother's repeated requests to come as soon as she could, so much so that she told her she would fly in on Friday when the rates were cheaper. Grandma apparently had a habit of dying regularly so one could interpret Jessie's standoffishness as someone saying, "Yeah, yeah, I heard this all before." Turns out that Jessie was wrong, and although Grandma pleaded, she couldn't get her daughter to budge.

So, Grandma died without the benefit of seeing her second daughter.

I didn't see my great grandma on the day she died. For some reason DeeDee decided that she needed to see great grandma that day and thought my mom should go with her. They arrived early in the am on May 15, 1981, and for the better part of the day their grandma slept. My aunt took Mom home and returned to find a rather somber scene. DeeDee was told that it looked as if my great grandmother had just died, that maybe she should go in *and check* as well.

DeeDee went into the room, and sure enough there was

great grandma, quiet and lying as if asleep, only she was dead. Her breathing had simply stopped, her heart followed, Great grandma had left as peacefully as anyone could wish for.

As sad as death is, I am not so sure that it truly is the end of things. Not long after she died the zaniness that surrounds my family began. My mother's father, John (Jack to all, and the man my son Jonathan is named after), awoke from his own trance-like sleep, stepped into the dining room and promptly sat at the table. All of the requisite calls had been made by my grandmother shortly before my mother and aunt returned to the house. Two of New York's Finest were in the house along with mom, aunt, grandmother and an obviously very dead great grandma, a curly haired Irish setter named Brandi, and...

...Jack, sitting at the table in his pajamas tapping his fingers and not saying a word. My mom gave a somewhat bewildered look to my aunt as if to say, "What the hell is *that* all about?" One would think that having two cops in the room would indicate that *maybe* something was wrong, but Grandpa sat there looking at the clock, tapping his fingers and looking rather annoyed.

My late grandfather was a life-long Navy man and probably the most ridiculously routined individual I have ever met. Looking at the clock my mother realized that it was precisely 5:15 p.m., and police in the house or no it was dinner time. There he sat awaiting the evening meal. Not knowing exactly what to say, and everyone in the house awaiting the coroner to officially do what my aunt had done hours previously (declare Katherine dead, as if her cold body wasn't an indication?), my mother said, "Daddy, *What* are you doing sitting there, Grandma died in the other bedroom!"

"It's five fifteen, and it's dinner time."

My mother, who by this time was furious at her own father went into the kitchen, threw together a ham and cheese sandwich and glass of milk for him, dropped the now made meal on the table and went back to waiting with everyone else.

Grandpa still sat there tapping his fingers not saying anything. He looked at the sandwich yet didn't make a move or take a bite. Now, both my mother and Diane looked at each other puzzled. It was then that DeeDee realized there was *ham* on the sandwich.

No meat on Fridays! Now you need to understand that Jack wasn't religious at all, so the mere fact that he refused meat on a Friday is hilarious by itself. When DeeDee realized what the problem was she reminded my mother who promptly said, "Look, the Pope in *Rome* is eating frigging ham, and if it's good enough for him it's good enough for *you!*"

Still there was no movement from him until my mother ripped the meat of the sandwich and threw it in the garbage. As soon as she was finished, without so much as a word being spoken, he quietly ate the cheese sandwich, washed it down and went into his room.

As he slipped into his room my mother made a remark, "When the coroner comes make sure that he goes into the right bedroom. When he sleeps, he looks deader than she does!" As a Navy man, and being on ships most of his adult life, he slept with his arms across his chest and straight. When he slept he didn't move. Mom wanted to make sure that they took the right person to the morgue.

Shortly thereafter, the coroner arrived, the police left and Great Grandma was finally moved.

Aunt Jessie and her husband, Jack, had decided to fly to New York on the very Friday great grandma died to save on the airfare. On a cloudless, beautiful and flawless day, her plane circled the city for almost four hours. One would have to think that since she couldn't come when asked, Great Grandma decided to make her daughter's life a little harder. I can hear her voice saying, "That'll teach you, Jessie. Have a nice landing."

Long into the day great grandma died, Jessie arrived to find out she was too late.

Funerals tend to be somber gatherings as family mourns the loss of their loved one and friends remember the decedent in a variety of ways. As mournful as the funeral home can be, great grandma was ninety. She had lived a full and interesting life, so not many tears were shed in sadness. People offered condolences to my grandmother and my aunts, and many neighbors and friends from the old building on Amsterdam Avenue came to pay their final respects.

The day of the funeral started like any other day. The sun was up and bright and I had to put on a suit jacket and tie (which I hated then, and hate *now*, twelve years of Catholic school will do that to a guy). Everyone else was all dressed up for the final goodbye and burial of grandma, as well.

My father, a month earlier, had purchased a brown Lincoln Mark IV from his friend Emil. Dad loved that car. Long and powerful with a 454 engine and four barrel carburetor, the Lincoln was as strong as it was sexy. I loved riding in it as it was smooth and quiet and it always smelled of leather. We piled into the car and made the long drive into Manhattan to 72nd Street for the final viewing before they closed the lid for the funeral mass.

Many floral arrangements surrounded her casket, and as funny as it sounds (and someone always says it, so let it be me this time), she looked peaceful, asleep. If I didn't know she was already dead, I would have guess that she had fallen asleep and would wake up from her nap shortly. The small casket (she was barely 5 feet tall, *maybe* in shoes) was oak and she had on a vintage dress from sometime in the early 1930's. In the middle of the flowers was a large arrangement of roses courtesy of my Uncle Jimmy, who was DeeDee's husband.

For years, Great Grandma attended mass daily but sometime later in life she had a falling out with the Roman Catholic Church. Her daily walks to mass ended. After waiting for hours for a priest to arrive to lead prayer service on the last night of the wake, it became apparent that none was going to show. The funeral director, who looked like a taller version of Bela Lugosi, called the church enquiring when the priest was coming.

Ordinations of new priests just happened to be on that day, and someone along the way had lost track of time. No priest was available. It was up to our favorite funeral director, Bela, to come to the rescue; he led the prayer service. When he was finished and the room remained quiet, he retired to the back of the room.

I am not exactly sure why Jimmy, my dad and distant cousin, Jay, were not on Grandma's favorite persons list but that day her revenge was exacted on each of them for transgressions I'm still not quite aware of. After the service, and as Bela walked to the back of the room, there was a loud *thud*.

My mom jumped, and audible gasps resonated throughout the small chapel as we turned to investigate the noise. I was hoping Great Grandma didn't decide to get up and in doing so knock the casket over. Much to my relief, she was still quietly laying in the coffin. What wasn't standing was a large floral arrangement, in the middle of a row! It was almost as if someone kicked the stand closed and the flowers tipped forward.

As we picked up the arrangement, we saw the ribbon attached to the top: *BELOVED GRANDMOTHER.*

On the card read the hand written words: "Love Jimmy."

One has to wonder if a small, spirited foot belonging to one Katherine Binnie kicked over the flowers as if to say, "Keep 'em!"

Great Grandma was never one to let a grudge go, and even in death she made her disapproval known.

After the final prayers were said, we went downstairs to get into the car and right away we saw that something wasn't right. As we walked toward the car, a noticeable puddle had formed and a long river of slick fluid was running toward the sidewalk. Dad popped the hood open and saw, much to his surprise, that in the area of the water pump, large volumes of antifreeze and water were pouring out! There was no way the Lincoln Mark IV, his pride and joy, could be driven. In a fit of rage (and to the snickers of my grandmother and aunt), he went to a payphone to call for help. Great Grandma, who did *not* like my dad at all, had made it abundantly clear that he wasn't welcome at the church, and she made *sure* he couldn't get there.

Soon after a tow truck carted the Lincoln away, Dad hopped a train to Queens to get his boss's Cadillac, and we got into DeeDee's van to go the half mile to the church.

However, lucky cousin Jay was having car problems as well. Jay, had lost favor with great grandma years before, yet he decided to come as family should and pay his respects to her. Jay owned vintage cars and was a good mechanic as well. He was meticulous in the care of all of his autos. Great Grandma didn't want him around either, and when he turned the key to start the car...

...*Nothing. Nada. Zilch. Zero. Donut!* The car was dead.

Dad's car had already gone, and with what Jay described as a dead battery (how fitting is *that*, a dead battery at a funeral!), we needed to jump start Jay's vintage Cadillac so we could get moving. No one had a large enough battery to do the job until the funeral director came up with a novel idea. He pulled the hearse along side of Jay's car, hooked the cables from battery to battery and jump started the car.

Inside of the hearse, with flowers on her casket...was Great Grandma. Probably laughing her ass off!

Situated between 59th and 60th Streets and Columbus Avenue in Manhattan, St Paul the Apostle church is a magnificently beautiful Gothic style church. Inside on the ceiling is a mural of the sky. If one looks up at night, it's as if the service is being held under a starry sky. My parents, aunt and various family members had been married in the church, and it was the place chosen to say the final mass for Great Grandma.

A very tired priest awaited us as we finally arrived en masse. There were a few small problems though. As magnificent an edifice as it is, St. Paul's echoes hollow when the organist forgets to come for the mass. The lack of incense was also an indication that this mass was going to be quick and to the point.

DeeDee had purchased a digital watch not too long before grandma died, and one of the features it possessed was a loud alarm. My cousin Michael, all of about two years old at the time, was playing with the watch in an effort by his parent's to keep him busy as the mass moved steadily along. There was no organ music, as there usually is at funerals, and I think grandma was bit pissed at the fact that the organist blew off her mass.

As the priest finished a short sermon and we were about to stand, Michael hit the correct button. The watch started playing "*I wish I was in the land of cotton...*" Dixie! As they scrambled to disable the watch and as an electronically poor rendition of Dixie echoed off the walls of the church, my grandmother says out loud, "Serves them right for not having an organist here. Ma always loved organ music!"

Great Grandma wanted music at her funeral, and in her own way, she got it.

At the very end, and over the gravesite, the final prayers were said and my great grandmother was *finally* laid to rest. She has been gone for almost twenty-eight years. I have had four of my own children, became a nurse and have had an interesting life myself. As I write this last testament to my

Great Grandmother, I hope that when I finally die and meet her again she won't be too mad at me.

I have a feeling that if she is, instead of a funeral dirge and a hearse I'll arrive at the church via Federal Express to a small band playing Dixie.

How fitting.

Death Isn't the Worst Thing

As I have moved through my career as an RN, I have seen many things. I have seen miracles and tragedies, illness and death and everything in between. The job of the nurse involves much more than just taking care of an immediate issue. Most times it involves taking care of the family as well. Patients who are ill often depend on the nurse to answer questions they either couldn't get answered by the doctor, or they were simply to afraid or intimidated to ask. I often get questions such as: "Will I ever get better? What will happen after I leave here? Can you validate my loved one's parking pass?" My job is to answer to the best of my ability, and most times I have an answer right away. And yet, there are times when I don't have one at all.

Part of being a nurse involves dealing with those life and death issues that arise and how to talk to and care for families as their loved one is dying. As sad as any death is, I can say with a great degree of confidence that there truly are things worse than the ultimate destination for all of us.

Suffering, to me is probably the worst thing I witness on an almost daily basis. Everyone I suppose has their own definition of suffering, but to me I try to be as pragmatic about it as I can. Horrible physical or mental pain is suffering and each of us has our own defined parameters as to what our own pain actually is. When I saw Michael just before he died, I saw suffering. I saw suffering in another friend as she dealt with her own cancer pain, and I was virtually powerless to do anything for her until the medication took over.

I have seen so many people suffer in so many ways. As the person ultimately in charge of their care, it was and is my job to make sure that the pain in any form goes away, or at least hides in a closet for a while. Narcotics serve a great purpose when used as they are intended (as pain medications they work extremely well, people abuse them for the side effects). Morphine in particular is one of the best. Morphine not only gives excellent pain control, but it also acts as a euphoria agent, often allowing the person to forget that the pain was there at all.

I remember when I was just a fledgling ICU nurse and had my first experience with a medicated Morphine drip. I was taking care of a patient affectionately known as Rico Swavay (spelled phonetically on purpose, and named after the song of the same name) in the ICU of a large metropolitan hospital in New York City. I learned a lot about caring for the suffering family as well as the patient, and I learned a tremendous amount about myself as a nurse because of him. Here is his story.

Rico was a patient who had long term liver disease resulting from exposure to Hepatitis C. He had been hurt in an industrial accident some twenty years before and as a result required multiple blood transfusions. One of those transfusions resulted in exposure to Hepatitis C and he became very ill as the virus attacked his liver. Eventually, after battling the virus for years, his liver began to shut down. He wound up on our transplant service awaiting a new one.

Rico prided himself on how well he looked even when ill, and his family was constantly at his side. He had two daughters and a wife who doted on him; they sat in his room day and night hoping that their presence would help motivate him to get better. They took turns in shifts and it was a wonderful experience to see how deeply the women most important to him loved and honored him even on those days when he was so confused he didn't remember who they were.

Each day they came, they combed his hair, talked to him and encouraged him to get better and come home. Questions came rapidly from them daily as they anxiously awaited word as to when an organ might become available. Each day he became more jaundiced despite the treatments we gave him. It was clear that very soon, if no organ was found, Rico would die.

I was caring for him in the unit one day and for the better part of the shift, he slept. One of the effects of high Bilirubin and Ammonia in the blood is severe confusion and lethargy. Rico's numbers were climbing higher daily and he was deteriorating steadily. His wife and daughters sat with him, talking to him about how well he would be after surgery, and not to worry that an organ was coming. Tears and crying were the norm in his close knit family. As I followed my two nursing rules, my concern for him and his family deepened.

My shift ran from 4 p.m. until midnight. One night just before I was about to leave, the phone rang. Rico now had a breathing tube hanging out of his mouth as he was very critical. I spoke to the surgeon on the phone and was told to begin the prep for the OR, that an organ had been found for Rico. He would be going to surgery at 5 a.m.

When I alerted his daughter, she jumped up out of her seat crying and called her mother. Within an hour, both of his daughters and wife were at his bedside holding his hand and telling him that his long wait was over.

Rico lay in the bed, intubated and not moving. As they cried tears of joy and I gave report to the oncoming nurse, the ICU was strangely alive with the sounds of the respirator, monitors and two nurses talking about the impending miracle surgery for Rico. All of us were happy and deep down I think Rico was jumping for joy with his family, although none of us could see it.

I went home that night, tired from another long day. As I lay in bed, I wondered how things would go and how Rico would be when I got back to work the next day. The surgery itself is long and intense, and the aftercare that follows is very structured with the nurses in the unit becoming very routined and methodical about care. As I dreamed, I thought about his family and how things would be after he was finally back in the unit and on the road to recovery.

The next day I arrived at work and found the scene to be much as I suspected. Rico was still in his bed, respirator whirring and monitors showing all of his life functions on a computer screen. There was a long line coming out of the right side of his neck called a Swan Ganz catheter, and he also had an internal bladder catheter, as well (also known as a Foley). His arms remained mildly restrained (to prevent grabbing and dislodging the breathing tube), and in his right wrist an arterial line gave us a true blood pressure reading.

His abdomen was a mass of bandages and drains, and medications dripped into him through the Swan in his neck and a second central venous line. The job now was to monitor everything and measure what was going into him and coming out, and to draw laboratory samples every few hours to monitor his new liver for function. His color still remained a dark brown and his eyes were yellow with *bilirubin*. His wife and daughters stood vigil over him, as usual. Now we were all waiting for the recovery phase to begin.

The one alarming thing I noticed right away (as did my fellow off-going RN) was that he wasn't really making enough urine despite the large volume of fluid he had received during the course of surgery and recovery. Kidney function and recovery are vital to the success of any surgery. The surgeons had been made aware of his situation before I came on shift. Various medications were used to try to make his body process the fluid and aid the kidneys in filtering and passing the urine out. His output was a deep, sickly brown, and we were alarmed.

So far, nothing was working.

Organ transplant surgery is an amazing thing to be a part of and watch through all phases. Generally speaking, when the patient arrives for the surgery, they are deathly ill and the surgery is the last resort. I have been a part of many liver and kidney transplants in my career, having been the receiving nurse as a newly transplanted patient returns and their road to recovery begins.

For the family, doctors and nurses, it is an exciting and stressful time. But as the patient gets better and they return to a normal level of functioning, the miracle that comes from the death of another makes the stress level less and sometimes results in a complete recovery. Then again, sometimes it doesn't.

Organ rejection is always a primary concern. As blood is drawn and analyzed the nurses and doctors can determine how the new liver is performing and whether or not rejection is happening. Medications are given usually immediately before the surgery to begin the long arduous journey to immune system suppression (a very crucial step in preventing the new organ from being attacked by the body's own defense system). Each and every day post operatively the same medications are given to make sure that rejection stays at bay.

I had cared for Rico well before his surgery and I knew him as well as I could before he slipped into the confusion of hepatic encephalopathy. (That term is the confusion related to toxins in the blood. As his liver failed, the Ammonia, which is a byproduct of protein metabolism overloaded the brain and he became lethargic and profoundly confused.) One of the hardest parts about being a transplant nurse is remembering the two rules, applying them, and remembering that not everyone is lucky and gets a new lease on life.

Then again, some do and the transplant isn't successful.

Over the course of my eight hour shift I adjusted medicated drips, gave large doses of diuretics (medications to help the kidneys get rid of excess water), and began the one drug I hated to give at all post transplant, steroids. Rico wasn't getting any better, in fact, he was getting worse. The intravenous steroids were being given in high doses in an effort to stem the rejection that was now obvious on his lab values.

When the consent for surgery was signed, Rico's wife and daughters were given every possible scenario regarding success and failure. When confronted with a life and death situation, most people that I have met choose life and want to try everything possible to fix whatever problem there is. Rico, before surgery, was extremely ill and his only chance was to transplant the diseased and dying organ in the hope that the body accepts the new one as its own.

In some cases, even after surgery, the body rejects the new organ and the patient dies regardless of everything done. (This is a perfect example of Rule #2.)

The vigil at his bedside continued for a few days, and it became abundantly clear that no matter what we did, the new organ was failing. The surgeon asked to speak to Rico's family about what to do next. I knew immediately what he was going to tell them. His family had been devastated once when he deteriorated and came to the ICU. They were so full of hope when the new organ became available, and now the surgeon had to give them the grim news that he didn't think that Rico would get better at all, that the surgery didn't work.

The one thing that concerned the family was Rico suffering any longer, and after a long consultation with all of the doctors involved, the decision to use a Morphine drip to ease his pain and help him feel as good as he could as he began the final journey home.

As Rico lay there it was plainly obvious to all of us that he had tremendous pain. He tried to shift himself and moaned periodically. When he was turned by one of us, he would wince and thrash. The pain had to be excruciating based purely on his reactions to how we moved him and his facial expressions. My direct supervisor (mentor, and to this very day the best nurse I have ever been around, what a distinct privilege it was to learn from her) came to me and said that we were going to start a Morphine drip per the family's request, and she wanted to go over the parameters with me.

The purpose of the drip was to allow Rico to be out of pain and help him become comfortable in the last days, hours, or minutes of his life. I had never used Morphine in that capacity and I was not very comfortable maintaining and increasing the drip as needed to help control his pain and suffering.

My supervisor, Barbara, and I sat down. We went over the protocol and use of the pump and lockout mechanism. My unique ID was the number used to track any changes in the dose and rate of flow, and she wanted to make absolutely sure I knew exactly what I had to do.

Rico lay dying, his body was now a twisted mess of tubes, surgery incisions and IV lines. His wife and daughters came into the room after speaking to the doctors. They approached me as I prepared the pump and drip for Rico. His breathing tube had been removed the day before and his respiration rate was now in the high fifties. He was taking quick, rapid, shallow breaths and was obviously struggling to breathe. He was in a tremendous amount of pain, as well. I spoke briefly with the three women and explained again as best I could what the drip was for and what the desired effect would be. Barbara was there, and when I was sure that the family and staff were on the same page, I hung the drip. I started the infusion at 1 mg an hour and waited.

Barbara sat there for the first half hour with me knowing that I was nervous about using the medication and lending support to the decision that the family made. One of the side effects of Morphine is a decrease in respirations. My concern was that he would be so decreased that it shut his breathing off completely. Rico was still not comfortable so I increased the drip to 2 mg an hour and continued to wait for results.

Barbara left and told me to page her with updates. The family sat the bedside continuing their vigil over him. His wife looked at me after another half hour had passed and asked me to increase the drip again as he was still so restless and uncomfortable. Per the protocol, I typed my ID in and increased the drip to 4 mg an hour.

And we all continued to watch Rico.

Still he struggled, and his breathing remained in the high forties. His daughters were each holding an arm and his wife was stroking his face telling him it was all okay now, that they would be fine and to please go to wherever he needed to go. They all told him to let go, that the family loved him and would miss him, but that his suffering needed to end. His breathing came in short pants, much as a winded athlete breathes after a long race or shift of ice time on a hockey rink (something yours truly can personally relate to).

I listened silently and struggled with the scene myself as it was heart rendering and touching to witness. I thought to myself how lucky he was to have a family who loved him so much that they *wanted* him to die so that the pain and illness he was suffering would finally come to an end. The girls were begging Daddy to please let go and stop suffering. The sobs coming from them were unbearable for me to hear.

I watched intensely as another half hour rolled past and Rico continued to writhe and moan. As soon as I was able, I increased the drop rate to eight mg an hour and went about monitoring his progress. His respiration rate dropped from the mid fifties to around forty. But even though the rate had dropped, he still was uncomfortable and was extremely restless.

I called Barbara when I increased the rate and asked her to please come speak with me on my dinner break. She told me she would be there shortly and to meet her in the conference room. I told her I would and got myself ready to leave for a well deserved half hour break.

I quickly gave my relief nurse an overview of what was going on and told her that I would change the drip rate if needed when I came back. Both of Rico's daughters had left to get something to eat themselves and his wife had her head on his hand in what seemed to be a prayer vigil.

I met Barbara in the conference room and gave her the latest news on how he was doing. She knew I was still struggling with things and she sat listening *again* about how I felt. I told her that I felt I was contributing to his death and that I was having an issue increasing the drip to 16 mg.

What she said to me made a profound difference in how I have approached life and death since that day in the ICU.

She told me to put myself in Rico's place, and asked what would I want?

"Not to be in pain, that's for sure", was the first thing I said.

"Mark, he is terminal. You are smart enough to understand what's happening and know that nothing more can be done. The family wants his suffering to stop. Whether he dies now, five minutes from now or five hours from now, don't you think that the best thing is be humane and make him as comfortable as you can? You can't kill someone with humanity, Mark. What you can do is treat him as best as you can given what you know, and make the last hours as pain free and comfortable as humanly possible. You need to increase the drip and not worry about *how* things look. Remember that you are the nurse in charge of making sure he is getting what he needs to be comfortable and pain free. If that was you there, what would you want your family to tell me to do?"

As I listened to her words, I realized that she was right. Both rules applied here: he was one of those patients who got sicker and was going to die, and nothing I knew or did would ever change the fact that he was going to die. So, I did what I would want someone to do for me in my time of dying, in pain, and suffering unbearably.

I went back into the ICU and turned the drip rate to 16 mg.

His wife and daughters continued to support and talk with him, and I watched to see if anything changed. Over the course of an hour his writhing slowly dissipated and his breathing pattern changed. The rate had gone from a panting breathless 52 to a more erratic but deeper 20. I checked his yellowed eyes for papillary response and found that they were pinpoint and not responding to my flashlight. His blood pressure had dropped and his heart rate was now in the fifties. Rico was quiet and deeply asleep, and I wondered how long he would continue to lie there. I called Barbara and told her of the status change. She told me she would be there soon.

I went over to the bedside with his family and pretended to be busy checking all of the lines. I asked his wife if I could do anything for them. She looked at me through swollen eyes and simply said, "No, Mark, you've already done everything. Rico really liked everyone who helped him; he especially liked how you spoke with him while he was sick the first time. Thank you."

I looked at both of his daughters to ask the same question and both shook their heads no. I glanced at the clock. It seemed like so much time had passed but it was only 7:15 in the evening. Barbara came down and read my running nurses notes. She looked at the monitors and his breathing pattern and wrote on a piece of paper, "I think it will be very soon. Maybe while you are here. If he changes call me right away."

She left the unit and I had a feeling that if she thought it was soon, that she was more than likely right. Shortly before 10:30p.m., I called her.

Over the passage of the next two hours or so Rico's breathing became labored. He wasn't writhing in pain, but his breathing pattern changed. He was having long deep breaths, followed by either a long pause or a burst of short rapid breaths. I knew that change was the sign that he was actively dying, and I could tell by how his family was reacting that they knew as well. His daughters were crying and saying, "Please Daddy, you can go now, I love you. Please, I'll be okay." His wife was whispering memories to him, reminding him of how they met and their wedding, and the births of their girls.

I watched as his heart rate slowly slowed down and his breathing became deeper with long pauses. With each pause, his heart rate dropped into the twenties and when he breathed it came back to around thirty-eight or forty. Finally I walked over the his bed when I saw the long pauses between heart beats and I stood next to his wife as she held his hand and said I love you one last time. The monitor started to alarm Asystole (otherwise known, my readers, as a flat line) and I quickly shut the volume off.

His wife and girls were with him holding his hand and I stood there trying to remain as emotionless as I could. When Barbara came into the room and I turned, she nodded at me.

Tears rolled down my cheeks and I left the room. That was the first time I actually watched someone just *expire*.

And as much as I hate to say it, it wasn't the last.

I suppose at the end of all this one would ask me how I feel some twelve years after this event. The truth of the matter is I went to a therapist for a few sessions to talk about what had happened and to validate my own feelings of using a Morphine drip for the first time, and to watch helplessly as my two rules of nursing unfolded.

I feel now that I did the right thing. If it was me lying there, I would want anyone doing for me, what I did for him. I acted as a good nurse should by considering everything about my patient and his family, their wishes and making sure that he was comfortable and pain free when he died.

I hope that when my time comes, someone takes the time to consider me lying there. After all, being human means caring for your fellow person.

Isn't that right?

Sometimes You Learn to Duck

Warm-ups before a game serve a few purposes. One reason to warm up is to allow your goalie to stretch out and face some shots so he can get into a save-making rhythm. Another is for guys to get their legs under them and start the initial flow of adrenaline that is needed to skate in a sixty minute contest. For me, warm-ups were a way to gather a little intelligence on the opponent and to watch their goalie go through his routine. If one knows a goalie's weaknesses one has a better chance at exploiting them

I usually went through a few minutes of stretching and my routine was to take exactly four shots on my own net. That allowed me to see where my aim was for the night and helped me gauge how I would shoot for the evening. However, I mostly skated slowly and methodically on my side of the center red line and watched the other team.

The Recreational League I joined in Florida was a mixture of some top tier players and guys just starting out. It was an eclectic mix of players and the teams were usually pretty even matched. My team, Yellow Snow (and yes, I picked the name as it suited me and my teammates perfectly), had a very good season and we were now in the playoffs. I skated on the first line on the left wing. My principal job was to score goals and on most nights I did.

My line mates were a lot younger than me and had the legs that I always lacked. Not blessed with breakaway type speed, my game was predicated on being in the right place at the right time and having line mates who required the other team to focus their attention on. Most of my goals were scored from ten to fifteen feet out in front of the net, and mostly on rebounds. For lack of a better word, I was the proverbial garbage man and for most of my playing days it suited me just fine.

Playing with guys a lot younger was a great experience. I always told people that I couldn't keep up with them all the time skating wise, but I could on the score sheet. On most nights we won, and our line of three was the top scoring line in the league. If my center or right wing scored, I was usually the one passing the puck. If I scored, it was either one or both of my line-mates who helped. We won a lot of games, and for the four years I skated with them, statistically speaking they were my best years.

I always set standards for myself at the beginning of the season. We played fourteen games then had playoffs in a round robin type tournament. Each season I set a twenty goal mark and for four straight years and three seasons per year, I hit that goal pretty easily. I loved playing hockey and as much as I miss it now, I won't skate in a game again.

All athletes get injured at one time or another. It is something that we all experience even on a low recreational level. Aside from some minor shoulder injuries and an occasional cracked rib (when you stand in front of the net and get pounded, that happens), I was pretty fortunate. I had been on the ice when a friend on another team took a quick turn, caught a rut and tore his knee to shreds. I can still hear the *pop* as the ligaments pulled off the bone and remember his scream as he grabbed his leg. Injuries are never fun and as hard as everyone plays and as much as you dislike the other team when competing, no one ever wants to see another guy hurt. When someone goes down you remember that it could have been you.

Sometimes in hockey you have to duck. When playing full contact in upper level leagues, body checks and sticks can come up high in the head area, so you learn to ultimately have eyes in the back of your head. You learn to respect the ability of the other players and be completely aware of everything going on around you. Sometimes things happen so fast that you duck just a little too late.

The first period started pretty routinely. We lined up at center ice, I did my usually ritual of tapping my opposing wingers shin guards and saying, "Have a good skate." We were playing the teal team this night, and I knew all of the guys as I had skated with most of them at one time or another. I was all warmed up and ready. The puck dropped and the game began.

The first few shifts were uneventful as each team gauged what the other had that night. The puck was in our zone and

I saw John, my center, break for an opening at the blue line. As he burst past two defenders, I put a perfect pass on his stick in mid stride and he went in all alone. One quick move and the score was 1-0.

In the last minute of the period John took the puck in our zone and skated through the middle. As two guys went to him, I was left open so that when the puck was left for me all I had to do was hit the net, which I did. I put my head down and fired without so much as looking at the goalie. When I didn't hear anything I knew it was in. At the end of one period we were up 2-0.

Midway through the second period the puck was going into our zone and I was skating as fast as this big body allows to retrieve the puck. Jay, the opposing player, was going as fast as he could, as well. When he fell in front of me and hit my legs, there was really only direction I could go.

There was probably eight to ten feet of room before I would hit the boards at full speed. I could see the boards coming straight at me. It seemed like time slowed down and I had a clear view of what I was about to hit head on. I was thinking *put your hands up* and just before I went head first into the boards, I did. I heard a sickening *THUD*, a crack and before I blacked out I thought the crack was my neck snapping. Then the lights went out.

About two minutes later I opened my eyes.

I was lying on my back moving my legs up and down, (good I thought, at least they move) and feeling like there was a hornets' nest inside of my head. My neck was sore, my helmet cracked and I had blood on my face where the skin on the bridge of my nose tore away from the collision. I was being asked who I was. When I said, "Dorothy, ain't this Kansas?" a small burst of nervous laughter escaped the players from both teams. I tried to get up and was wobbly so I was assisted back to the bench to collect myself.

That was a relatively funny way to look at it, my brain was mush. I sat at the end of the bench with my head in my hands and cleaning the blood of my face. I was asked repeatedly if I was okay, and of course I said, "Sure, I need a helmet."

I was able to get a helmet from one of the other guys waiting for their game, and when I put it on I sat at the end of the bench for a moment. My head was like lead, and my feet felt funny. The second period had ended and I climbed over the boards to see if I could skate. I took a few turns around the rink and in retrospect probably should have gone straight to the locker room. I knew that I was needed by my team and as bad as I felt I was stupidly determined to help win the game.

I played the rest of the game in a fog with a very slow reaction time. I watched video of it a few months later and wondered how the fuck I didn't end up with a broken neck. The sound of the impact was much like that of baseball bat hitting a cardboard box. Although I couldn't see much from the angle of the camera, I knew that I was lucky I could still walk.

I saw on video how a perfect pass came to me and after the puck passed me by, I reacted. As funny as it looked on the television screen, it really wasn't a funny thing to see. What I saw was someone who took a hard whack to the head and was showing the effects of it. It was scary to experience, and even more frightening to watch.

I did manage to drive home. By the time I got there everyone was asleep. I had already showered at the rink, so I propped some pillows under me (my neck was throbbing and I had a headache that would have killed a zombie) and tried to rest. Both of my eyes were blackened (I looked like an overly stuffed clownish raccoon), and I had a big cut between my eyes along the bridge of my nose. I settled down to sleep, which I did for about an hour.

Then, I had to run into the bathroom as the nausea and vomiting started. I knew what it meant, and it wasn't good. I was supposed to work in the morning at the stress test lab moving patients back and forth for their tests and keeping track of vital signs and the heart monitors. The one disadvantage to being an agency nurse was that I earned no sick or vacation time, so, if I missed a day of work I didn't get any compensation at all.

I decided to rest as much as I could before I had to go to work feeling as though my head was really a bag of cement. For lack of a better term, that is exactly how it felt.

My then wife was up early and when she looked at the raccoon eyes and spit nose she asked what happened. I told her I wasn't too sure but that I remember tripping over someone and hitting face first into the boards resulting in the damage she saw. She helped bandage my nose and said, "That's what happens when you play that dumb game. Are you leaving for work?"

I said, "Yes, I am already dressed. I'm fine."

"Do you think you might need a CT of your head?"

"Why, so I can pay all that money for them to tell me I have a concussion, I already know. My head feels like cement, my ears are ringing and I threw up all night. I gotta go." And soon thereafter I left for work.

Work that morning wasn't that busy. From the schedule I knew I would be done for the day by 1 p.m. I wasn't hungry and although my head was pounding, the nausea had subsided. The stress lab RN, Wanda, took one look at me and asked what did the other guy look like. Even though I laughed, it really wasn't too funny. I asked her a few times when we were starting to work and the look I got from her was all but saying, "Why did you even bother to come in?"

The answer to that question is simple actually. No work, no money, and I had four children and a household to support. The needs of the many certainly outweigh the needs of the one, don't they?

I got through day one and found myself fatigued and sick. I managed to sleep a bit when I got home; the kids had gone out for the day to a friend of their mother's. Over the course of the next week or so the nausea went away and gradually the hornets' nest in my skull subsided to just a few of the nasty buzzing insects. I looked less like a raccoon and began to be more of myself. I was constantly fatigued, but I went about my day as if nothing had happened.

I took the first five games off from the next season to make sure that the symptoms were gone. For the most part, when I returned for the first game, they were. I was glad to be back out on the ice that Friday; it was good to be among a group of guys I considered friends. I felt a step slower and my reactions were rusty, but all in all everything seemed fine.

Professional players such as Eric Lindros, Wayne Chrebet, Al Toon and Pat LaFontaine all suffered from what is called Post Concussion Syndrome. The syndrome itself is a relatively new term and it describes the feelings and symptoms of repeated blows to the head or the after effects of a hard hit. I can relate to all of them, and I must say I sympathize with any athlete who has suffered a bad knock to the head.

The problem is most secondary concussions aren't from a direct blow. They can result from simply running into an opponent and having your head snap as in a whiplash type of injury. Helmets are designed to prevent skull fractures and though newer helmets are very protective and well padded, they don't prevent concussions.

After the first concussion the chances of getting another dramatically rises and with each subsequent one it takes longer to recover. The aforementioned athletes all had to retire early due to the effects of multiple concussions, and I wish that somehow those injuries could be prevented by the design of a better helmet. The reality is this, it seems virtually impossible to prevent the brain from slamming into the skull, helmet or no helmet. It is a risk that we all take when we participate in a contact sport, and for most of us, nothing happens.

You might be asking yourself, *"Did it happen again and what now?"* Well dear reader, the answer is simple: Yes, it did. I didn't get the next one from a fall or a blow to the head, but as I was turning to go up ice I ran into my own teammate. My head snapped briefly and the dizziness returned. Nausea started that night and the constant buzzing in my head was an indicator that once more there was a problem. My short term memory started to change as I couldn't remember where I put things, or what day of the week it was.

I worked through it, took time off the ice again, and waited until the symptoms got better before I played again.

Six weeks later I started over and everything was fine. I got through the season until the playoffs for the fall campaign started right before Christmas in 2006. We were behind with a few minutes left to go when I scored to tie the score. As I looked up and turned, I ran into a player from another team and fell.

After that I don't remember much. I know I scored because I asked for the score sheet and took it home with me. The kids were at their mother's house, and I was alone in the small apartment I rented. When I put the hockey bag away for the last time it was kind of a somber feeling. But then I remembered why it is that as parents we make the decisions that we do.

My life and the lives of the children are more important than playing a game. I had a job and children that lived with me to care for. Hanging up the skates and equipment was easy.

But I can say this, not too long ago I put my skates back on. I could feel the ice as I cut and circled the clean smooth surface. I could taste the crispness in the air and smell the ice as I turned around the rink. It was exhilarating.

There is this itch inside of me that I cannot quite scratch. When I'm on a rink just skating, I can think and not have to worry about anything. I think of all the goals I scored, all the games I played, all the nights when I hurt from giving a maximum effort and I mostly think of how I loved every minute of it.

I also remembered this: Sometimes you duck too late.

I'll watch games and skate with the kids. As for the old equipment bag, it will stay where it is now: in my dad's garage packed full of memories.

As much as I loved it all, I don't want to duck anymore.

It Happens When You Least Expect It

All nurses have memories of certain patients they have cared for, and I am certainly not an exception to any rule. Most memories are positive and when patients who are terribly ill manage to turn around and get better, it makes my job worth it.

Going through any nursing program is difficult. It takes a lot of dedication and perseverance to muster the strength and determination to actually finish. My class in Lehman College started at well over one hundred students in early 1991. By the time the program was complete there were around 60 or so. Some left of their own volition and others couldn't make the grades to graduate. Only the best and strongest survived.

For me nursing was a second career. I was able to work in a back office, Wall Street job in the mid 80's while I went to school at night. I graduated with a Bachelor's Degree in Economics, and since I worked in corporate library services, the degree helped me better understand how things are in the business world. A mere six months after receiving that degree, I decided to work on a Bachelor's in Nursing. Going back was a very smart executive decision.

I passed the boards in September of 1994 and began work as an RN in early 1995 in the transplant unit of NYU Medical Center in Manhattan. Orientation was an experience in itself. Finally after eight weeks in the classroom and on the floor with a more experienced nurse as a guide, I was able to take a full load of patient's on my own and practice as an RN. I had waited a long time to do so. Each day was not only a learning experience but brought new challenges and knowledge to me.

The mentors I had there were the best nurses I have ever worked with. Each of my mentors (there were three) taught me a little differently and shaped me as a nurse so that when I eventually went on to manage a unit a few years later, I was able to use what each of them left with me. Having any of them around was always a good thing, and in an emergency situation I usually deferred to their experience. As I gained more knowledge and skills I was trusted more and after 9 months I asked to be trained to the ICU.

And I was.

Working in the liver transplant ICU was probably by far the best learning experience I have ever had. Not only was I trusted to receive a fresh post operative patient, but I was allowed to think and reason as well. Very strict protocols were in place for the nurses to follow based on his or hers judgment and evaluation. It was demanding and exciting all at the same time and the sickest people I ever took care of came through that unit. I saw miracles there.

I also saw tragedy as well.

One night I was caring for a stable, post operative patient who was past the need of the ICU and was getting ready for transfer to a Step Down Unit. I had given report to one of the nurses on my floor and was packing the patients belongings when my supervisor said we were getting a transplant service patient in a few minutes with a variceal bleed. We cleared the transferring patient quickly and got ready for what was going to be a rough time. Variceal bleeds are usually horrendously bad and bloody.

A varicie is a tortuous, stretched blood vessel usually in the esophagus (food pipe, if you are unaware) on into the stomach. They are the direct result of severe or end-stage liver disease; when they burst the results can be devastating. A person with varicies is usually a walking time bomb. At the point of which this story is being told, I had been a witness to one severe bleed. All indications were that this one was as bad and that the patient was very critical.

The patient (name changed to George for obvious reasons) was a forty-one year old man being brought in after sitting down at his table to eat and vomiting a large amount of blood before he passed out on his floor. EMS had been quickly called and he was rushed to the nearest medical center in Brooklyn. He had been given a large amount of blood and had what was known as a Blakemore Tube inserted to try to put pressure on the varices that had erupted. When a patient with a Blakemore came into the ICU, it was usually not good at all.

The patient arrived at 8:45 p.m., and the blood bank had been notified to have a large volume of O negative blood and plasma ready for him. The Blakemore, a long red rubber tube was in his nose and each of the balloons on the inside was inflated to pressurize the still bleeding blood vessels. He was unconscious, as expected, with dried, blackened blood around his mouth and nostrils. He was extremely pale and the team was ready to intervene as best we could.

The one good thing about him, (which at this point is hard to believe that *anything* could be good) was that the other hospital placed a deep central venous IV into him already. That made getting blood into him a whole lot easier. Two nurses and doctors were at the bedside and each of us had a specific task. Two nurses checked the blood products for accuracy, one nurse ran the infusions, one documented, one circulated around getting supplies, the chief surgeon gave the orders and the residents placed new lines we needed. My job was to make sure that everything ran smoothly and assist as needed, and to infuse the blood once it became available. He was bleeding to death as he came into the room.

Crimson red was flowing around the tube and out of his mouth as we transferred him over to the bed. Units of blood were quickly checked and were handed to a nurse who was standing on a stool and infusing it as fast as she could. A ventilator was breathing for him. The goal now was to stabilize George as fast as we could. Each minute that went by seemed like an eternity as blood and plasma (which contains the much needed clotting factors he lacked) were squeezed in as fast as we could hang them. A Gastroenterologist (a specialist of the GI tract) was quickly getting his scope ready in an attempt to look for and possibly seal off the source of bleeding.

I was assisting with the scope. As the doctor carefully guided it in and saw the carnage that was inside, he rapidly began the process of using what is termed *Sclerotherapy*, which is physically using a chemical to seal off the bleeding. He asked me to quickly turn George.

We did, and a fountain of bright red blood poured out of him onto the floor. It looked like a war zone.

His vital signs were horrible, he had almost no blood pressure and his heart rate was in the high 120's. We just kept doing our best to save him, pumping in blood as fast as we could. I was covered in blood and thought to myself that the gown and three pairs of gloves I put on was smart. Although my clothes were protected, my shoes weren't covered by anything. By the time we were done, I was down one pair of Nikes.

We did eventually stabilize George; it was a collective effort from all of us. He had three varicies that bled, but the doctor was able to staunch the flow, and the twenty-eight units of blood we gave him were enough to keep him stable.

The next ICU nurse received shift report from me and I went home a bloody mess and exhausted. I tossed my shoes in the trash and took a shower for what seemed like an hour. I couldn't get the smell of the blood off me, no matter how much I washed.

You may be asking yourself, after all of that, what happened next? Well, when I got back to work the next day (in a pair of brand new shoes at a cost of $100), I learned all about George from the off going nurse.

George had been a heavy drinker for over twenty-five years, which meant that he started somewhere in his early teens. He dabbled in IV drugs years before and contracted Hepatitis C, (which made me thank my maker more that I gowned and gloved as I had). He had been clean for almost three years and was eligible for a transplant. He lay in the bed chemically sedated with a machine blowing life into him. He was still receiving blood product although his labs were improving slightly. He wasn't out of the woods yet, but he was stable.

George lay in the ICU for three weeks until finally he was stable enough to be moved out into a step down unit (a unit for four beds to one nurse. He was still serious, but not at death's door as previously). He was weak, but walking and feeling better. We were keeping a watch over his ammonia level (a product of protein metabolism) to make sure he didn't begin the slow painful decent into confusion. As the days post ICU wore on the battle to keep his ammonia level down was getting more difficult and he began to get confused.

Then he began to get violent with the staff.

One of the hardest parts about being a nurse is when they have to make the decision to use any kind of restraint.

Chemical restraint is the use of different agents to sedate or effectively calm a patient down. Often it takes a combination of different medications. Physical restraint is just as it sounds: the use of restraining devices that anchor to the bed to keep the patient from harming him or herself and others. George came back into the ICU restrained to the bed awake, angry and confused.

There were a few options I had to choose from, neither one was really any better than the other so I took the path of least resistance first. I spoke with him, reminding of him who I was, where he was and why. I also told him that the restraints had to stay on as long as he was violent or a threat to himself. Having a patient call me an asshole, or say, "Fuck you," doesn't bother me since sometimes I expect it, and as nurses we all face verbally abusive patient's at one time or another. When he spit at me across the room and continued to do so, my decision became easier.

I decided to use a medication to calm him down. Following the pre-set protocol, I gave him a small dose and waited. Over the course of two hours he was still screaming and cursing, so I gave him a little more each time until he calmed down and began to sleep. Once he was asleep I undid his arm restraints and let him rest.

George became more restless and confused as the days wore on. He remained in the ICU undergoing different treatments to keep his liver and body functioning until a new organ could be found. The nurses and doctors battled with electrolyte imbalances, high toxic ammonia levels and ever increasing bilirubin levels. Another breathing tube was inserted when he his respiratory status became compromised. George became sicker, and no matter what we did, he was dying a slow, agonizing death.

About a month after he got to the hospital and after countless battles with different medical complications and George hostilities, something wonderful happened. He went to surgery, received his new liver and came back to me fresh out of the operating room. The long battle he began many weeks prior seemed to be coming to an end.

George did well the first few days after surgery. His breathing tube came out on his third day post op and his liver was functioning as well as could be expected. His color was getting much better from the deep jaundice that he had and his mental status was much improved. We were able to get him well enough to transfer out to the step down unit next door. The great thing about all of this was he was getting much better.

There were no children; the only visitor George had was his wife. She had suffered with him through all of his previous battles with illness and had been his only real support system other than the doctors and nurses. Our unit was unique in that the patients and their families became close to the staff. We all understood our professional boundaries but there were many times I sat on the edge of a bed and just listened as the patient or family talked. It was my job to listen, and when they were done offer advice or console them as best I could. As an outsider looking in, I suppose they thought it was easier to have me listen to whatever problem they had and try to solve it for them.

It was great seeing the results after surgery. George was feeling as if he had a new lease on life. His wife was very happy at how well he was doing and it was almost time for him to be discharged. I went home for the weekend thinking it was the last time I would see him as a patient. I have to tell you that is actually one of the best feelings I can have as a nurse. When my patient goes home healthy it makes all of the trials, tribulations and hard work worth it.

I came back Monday to find that George hadn't left after all. He was walking around the unit Saturday morning when he felt dizzy and fainted. His heart monitor showed a dangerously low heart rate and the medication they gave him to try to increase the rate didn't work. He was having severe chest pains and he was rushed back into the ICU. Tests revealed that he had a heart attack. He was again critical.

Over the course of the next week George walked that fine balance beam between recovery and disaster. In the end he recovered. The decision to place a permanent pace maker was made because George still had bouts of dangerously low and erratic rhythms. With the device in place it could control the speed at which his heart beat and control the rhythm, as well.

The pacemaker was inserted and George did very well. He was up walking the next day, and since his new liver was functioning well, the decision to discharge him was made for the end of the week, Saturday morning! Everyone was excited, the doctors and all of us nurses were ecstatic that finally he was well and going home.

He had been with us for a little over four months total, and at one time or another all of us had cared for him. Some like me watched as his life walked the razor's edge, others took care of him on the general floor. His wife came in to take his belongings that Friday night, and they asked to see me on my dinner break.

There was a nurse from another unit named Sara in charge of his care that evening. I told her that I was entering the room and would be out shortly. Only he was there and as I walked in he stood up and said he wanted to tell me something. I said, "Sure, go ahead. What's on your mind?"

"We've been through a war together, man. A lot of times I was so out of my mind and nasty, and I wanted to say, thanks! If it wasn't for you and everyone in the ICU the first few nights, I'd be dead. I can't say enough." With that, he grabbed me in a bear hug and was sobbing on my shoulder.

I told him that he was finally getting to go home, the one place he wanted more than anything. He said he sure was, and I used my "Good thing you have ruby slippers, man" line on him. We both chuckled. Before I left I asked him how he was feeling and he said, "Other than this weird pain in my back, pretty good. The doc gave me some Percocet, but it really isn't working."

I thought quietly to myself for a second and said, "You know it might be muscular pain, George. You were in bed for a long time so that seems pretty logical."

He laughed and said, "I feel like I'm being paroled again." I shot him a look and we both laughed out loud.

The last thing I said to him was, "George, stay well and the next time you come back, make it for a visit, ok?"

"You got it man; I don't ever want to be looking up at you guys from a bed again, *ever*."

No more prophetic words were ever spoken by someone.

I had turned and walked out of the room and was heading for the nurses' station when I heard his nurse, Sara, scream for help and run out of his room. She was screaming for the code team. I ran back in.

On the bed was George, gasping like a guppy out of his bowl and foaming at the mouth. I quickly assessed him and felt no pulse. His breathing was all wrong. Short gasps were coming out of him and he wasn't moving *any* air at all. I grabbed the ventilation bag off the wall and began feverishly squeezing air into his lungs. His eyes were rolled into the back of his head and I was screaming for help.

Sara came in with the crash cart and soon everyone else came into the room. Sara took over bagging him and I started CPR. The code team came in and took over running the code although I was staying and giving CPR for as long as I needed to. There was no way I was leaving the room.

We worked at a frenetic pace. My shoulders were aching from the compressions and I was out of breath. I felt the sweat running down my back in little rivulets; my eyes were burning with tears. Orders were barked out by the resident in charge and my boss Barbara was running the medications one by one in rapid fire succession, we defibrillated (shocked) his heart numerous times. Still the monitor showed a ventricular arrhythmia called *v fib*.

We kept working on him, doing everything we could and still nothing. Some of the girls were crying and I was pumping as hard as I could, and still nothing was working. Forty minutes after we started the transplant surgeon arrived in a tuxedo; he had been out with his wife at a fundraiser somewhere in the city.

The doctor looked at George. George's pupils were open like two huge black saucers, and then we all looked at the monitor. The doctor saw the same thing we did, v fib with pacing spikes. (That is the line on the monitor that shows that the pacemaker is shocking the heart to beat.) He asked what we had done. We were still working on him, and I was exhausted and sweaty. The recording nurse quickly gave him a report of all we had done, and he said to stop.

I did stop. I already knew a long time before, but I kept working because I hoped that what I knew was wrong. We had walked a tightrope for so long, and now he had tumbled into the ravine below. I was breathing hard, and hot tears rolled down my cheeks.

"He's gone, folks," the surgeon said. "This is a simple case of a pacemaker failing. I cannot believe you guys missed this. No one was here when this happened, how long was he *down* before you found him?"

The silence in the room was broken only by the soft crying of some of my colleges and the hard breathing of me. I was furious at what I had just heard.

You have to understand that inside every person is someone that is buried. Someone that no one sees, nor should they. Deep down, in the furthest reaches of the soul lurks this beast we all have. I have this gate inside of me that remains closed unless, as was the case here, I get so pissed off that the dragon which lurks behind it roars and spits fire. I felt the rage and sadness inside of me boil, and out flew the dragon without a warning or regard for those who stood in his way.

"*MISSED*? How *long* was he down *for*?" I screamed. "Tell me, just who the *fuck* are *you* to come here from a *party* and tell anyone that they weren't *here*?" My boss told me to stop but I kept on going, I figured if I'm going to lose my job it should be for a good reason.

"Don't you *dare* tell me we weren't here. I was in this room not ten seconds before this happened. He hugged and kissed me goodbye then went down, and I *wasn't* here? You weren't. Pacemaker failure, my ass. Don't you come in here and tell anyone we missed anything. The only thing *MISSED* was the fact that as the surgeon on *CALL*, you were out with your wife at some fucking party. We were all here, and as far as I can see, you weren't."

My boss put her hand on my shoulder in an effort to calm me down. That made it worse. "Don't touch me, *AT ALL*. I don't need this shit from him or anyone here."

And I stormed out.

About fifteen minutes or so after George was declared dead, I was sitting in the ICU alone, still sweaty and shaking. What had just happened? He just turned and died, and I had no idea why. The surgeon and my boss walked in, and I knew what was coming.

I looked up at both of them, red faced and eyes puffy. The surgeon said to me, "Look I was upset, you were upset. I don't know what just happened. I walked in and he was already dead. I'm sorry that I said anything. I think I was wrong."

"Yeah, well, you know doctor, I was wrong for spouting off. The man just said 'thanks' and 'goodbye' and I watched him die not five minutes after. We did what we could, it didn't work." My boss didn't say anything at all, she just stood there.

"Everyone did a good job, all of you. Thank you for your hard work. We will post him (do an autopsy), and we'll see what happened."

"He said he had this weird back pain for a few days. That was all he said to me." I said as he turned and left the room.

I cleaned up and went back to caring for patients, and when it was time for someone to take George to the morgue, I took him.

All I said as I put him in the morgue was, "I'm sorry, we tried."

I didn't sleep that night, or the night after. I kept seeing his face begging me to help him and the last guppy-like breaths rolling out of his foamed encrusted lips. I still see that time to time when I have nightmares.

A few days later after the dust had settled and I could actually look my supervisor in the face again without feeling like a total schmuck, the report came back on George.

He wouldn't have survived that episode no matter who was there. He didn't die from a malfunctioning pacemaker, or from a heart attack. That back pain he was complaining about? The grafted artery in the new liver was leaking slowly, causing his pain. We never considered that possibility because he had been out of surgery for so long. In retrospect, I learned a valuable lesson that day. Back pain in a transplant recipient can be an indication of bleeding. I never forgot that, and that memory served me well a few times later in my career.

Essentially, the main artery to the liver broke open and he bled internally. Nothing we did would have prevented his death; he was essentially dead when I started compressing his heart. His blood volume was in his abdominal cavity and since he wasn't getting oxygen to his brain and other organs, they quickly died one at a time.

We coded him for fifty-two minutes, and in reality it was about forty-eight minutes too long. George was gone as soon as that artery broke open and poured his life's blood out into his belly. We didn't miss anything that day.

Everything just happened when we least expected it.

Memories of Time Past

People often ask me how it really is to finally be home. While it seems simple enough to answer, for me is actually rather difficult. Leaving Florida was tough because I tried to make a life there, and, for a time, I did. I left friends behind, people whom I valued and have missed since I took the kids up the coast in December of 2008. I left behind a life that I thought would be better. I guess making that executive decision wasn't as easy as I would have liked.

The best thing I could have ever done for the kids and for me personally was to do what I did: leave and come back to where I knew my home was and had always been. A very dear friend once told me that home would always be waiting for me, and she was right.

The night we came over the bridge and I was able to see the lights of my city through the snow, I knew I was where we belonged. The kids settled in easily as daily routines and school made them better and stronger little people. The one thing I hadn't done was go back to where it all started for me. I did that recently and it was then that I knew I was really home.

I decided on a Saturday to put the kids in the car and just go for a drive. Often in Florida I would tell them we were going somewhere and we just get in the car and go. That Saturday was no different than any of the other trip we spontaneously went on. Once I drove over the long span of the Whitestone Bridge and headed toward the always crowded Cross Bronx Expressway, I knew where the car would lead me.

As if on some runaway magic carpet, the car was headed north. We went up and over Rosedale Avenue and onto the beaten road of the Bronx River Parkway. Years of cars trudging along the road left sunken tracks which led my car like a train to the Mosholu Parkway Exit. We were on autopilot and I watched the road as the car steered around the bend and past the Botanical Gardens and Twin Lakes, up past Allerton Fields where I played ball as a boy. Mosholu Parkway came into view and the next thing I knew we were turning past

Frisch Field and the 52 Precinct House and up onto the corner of Decatur Avenue.

That was where it all began.

Standing on the corner of Decatur Avenue and Mosholu Parkway was something I had done almost daily for twenty-eight years. I looked across the street and saw the park that I played baseball in as a kid, and when I closed my eyes I could hear my friends' voices through the wind that blew through the limbs of the dead trees. The many trees that once lined the park were almost all gone now, taken by a recent invasion of beetles or sawed down by the destructive force of an overzealous developer.

I could see the ramp which led from the park to the footpath along the parkway. Many nights as teenagers our gang of friends hung out there. Some of them smoked their first cigarette there; most of us drank small bottles of beer (affectionately known in my early years as *Nips*) and got drunk on weekends. Most nights we just sat there and talked and listened to music on an old beat up boom box. If one goes back there and listens through the wind and sounds of the cars as they pass, you can still hear that radio playing.

I walked north with my kids in tow, smelling the air and looking at the street I lived on, taking in the sites and remembering. I remembered the old Fein house and who lived there and just adjacent to it the six story apartment building in which two of my friends lived. I remembered delivering groceries there and thanking God that the building had an elevator. Trudging up the stairs with crates full of someone else's food was hard work.

I heard the echoes of voices I haven't heard in so long. I wish I could see their faces as well. I heard my old gang of friends, both boys and girls alike loudly announcing someone had been tagged or found in a game of manhunt. The summers were filled with long nights of street games and laughter. I saw the sewer cap that was second base in stickball and remembered using an old broom handle for a bat, hitting a Spaldeen ball long, high and hard into the air.

I also remembered the sound of the glass breaking when I took out a window on the 5th floor of one of the buildings. I think of how pissed off my mother was and how my father laughed when he heard that the ball I hit went through the glass and into the old lady's kitchen. Such wonderful childhood memories flooded into my head again. I longed to see my old friends.

My children were asking so many questions, curiosity was the word of day, but Daddy was strangely quiet. I walked past a six story building and passed the first floor apartment of a long lost friend. I remembered speaking to her and her siblings through that open window many years ago. The building remained as it was when I was young, though someone had power washed years of dirt and grime off of it. Surprisingly enough for an old building filled with the ghostly sounds of so many footsteps, it looked good.

I walked past the first apartment building we lived in and saw the old stairs my mom had sat on as she watched my sister and me in the street. I see my old friend Chris's apartment windows and now someone new lived there. It wasn't quite the same anymore as everyone that I knew had either moved on or, in some cases, passed on. Across the street lived another friend, Vinnie. I remember when he first got married and when his first son was born. I could hear my own voice calling up to the windows looking for them to come down so we could all go and ride bikes or play ball.

If I called out now no one would come, and the kids would think their dad had completely lost his mind.

I saw my old apartment on the fourth floor of 3070 Decatur and looked at my old window. I could see my long dead dog hanging out of it acting like the neighborhood watchdog. I could hear his barks and whines like I used to when he saw either me or someone in our family walking in the street. And I remembered all those years I spent there growing up with my family. I took a picture of the kids on the steps of that old building. An old Spanish lady who I didn't know looked at me as she started to walk past. My eldest said out loud, "My dad grew up here."

I don't think she understood English as she just smiled and moved on.

Next to my old building was Red Brick, a private house that served as both a meeting place and base of the variety of street games we played. Easily identifiable by the red brick porch, it served its purpose well. I could remember endless summer nights, the air hot and thick, playing street games such as Ring-A-Leevo and Manhunt for countless hours. There were many nights in my adolescence and teen years where there would be fifteen to twenty kids using that porch as a base until a team mate flew out and freed them from their captors.

I could think back clearly and remember the first real kiss I ever got was on that porch. I was fourteen years old and it was the middle of the summer in 1979. She was the first girlfriend I had. As awkward as it was, it is a lasting memory and one that will stay with me forever. The porch wasn't brick nor was red anymore. Many years ago, it was replaced with stone and mortar by the people who bought the house when the previous owner died. No matter, though. To me it will always Red Brick. I think if you ask anyone who lived there all those years ago, they would tell you the same thing.

Across the street was a string of private homes that housed many of the families I knew and grew up with. The Hoffmans had a three story private home with a parking lot. Three families, all related to each other, lived there for as long as I can remember. When I got my first real car, I parked there and often during the summer I was invited to swim in their above the ground pool.

I remember Jerry and his family and the home they had next to the Deluca and Moscardelli families. Other families such as Sardinia and Whelan lived there, though their children were older than my group. Seeing those homes so many years after I left brought memories back like flood waters.

The kids were quiet as we walked. I stopped near my friend Vinnie's old house and next to that the old D'Ambroisio home. Both on my side of the street, they were older style homes that I had been in on many occasions. The thing about those old places was that they each had such a rich history and past to them. As you walked up the old wooden stairs, they creaked under the weight of your feet. It was almost like being in a turn of the century wooden farmhouse. All of them had changed in some way, but as I looked at them I could see what they once were and who used to live there.

As kid we used to run through the interconnected yards separated only by small walkways or fences. I could still see my friends running and being chased in the endless pursuit games we played. Even though the old grape vines were long gone from behind the neighborhood's chain link fences, that nasty, tart taste from those grapes still sat in my mouth. We couldn't help it, we *had* to try them each year. I looked at the roof of the old shed my friend Mike fell off and broke his arm and shook my head, laughing silently. I could hear the owners yelling at us not to trample the flowers or tomato plants.

Those people were all gone now, replaced by strangers who had no idea what memories there were right in front of them. They couldn't hear the faded echoes of years past like I could. Faintly in the background, I could hear my mom calling me out of my bedroom window telling me that dinner was ready. No one could hear that but me, and no one should.

I passed the old Tangredi house, a large, one family structure owned by the grandfather of a long since lost friend. I remembered the old piano in the sitting room, and the long, winding stairs up to second floor. Outside was a large yard fenced in and home to a parking lot now. Back then, we used to run up the driveway and hop the fence to hide from whoever was chasing us. Sometimes we would just hide in our jungle. The bushes that were there covered us perfectly and we would wait until we were able to rush out and free our trapped teammates on Red Brick.

On our block was an old house owned by Mr. Stimphel. To look at it now with its yard stripped bare of the trees that once were there, it doesn't seem to be the imposing scare factory it was so many years before. Any one of the group of kids I grew up with would tell you that it was haunted, and I can't decide whether or not it was. At night its dark exterior was hidden in the shadows of the trees that surrounded it. Light almost ceased to exist there; it was always so gloomy and foreboding.

Not very long before I wrote this, I spoke to an old friend who I hadn't seen or heard from in years. I had posted some pictures from this trip down memory lane on a website, and when she saw them she remarked, "Oh my God, I remember that house. It was scary!" She was right; it was scary when we were kids. Now it's just an old house in my old neighborhood looking different and somewhat lonely. I think if it could talk, maybe it would ask where all of us kids had gone that it used to scare so much.

Well, one of them is right here, old house. I liked you better when you were scary and haunted. Now you are too open and your mystery is gone.

Time changes all things, though I thought I saw the hunched over image of old Mr. Stimphel as he navigated those old stone steps. I can hear the old wooden cane *CLICK* as he stepped. Maybe that house is haunted, Kathleen. Maybe.

I looked at the string of private homes that were across the street from the old Stimphel House. Starting at the Phillips house, I remembered many days of swimming in Walt's pool, which was by invitation only. When I grew up and was able to drive, I rented a parking spot from his aunt. It was a relief to have my car off the street. Next to Walt's old house was the Milky house, owned by a stooped over old man who's main task in life was to keep us kids out of his small front yard, and his flowers intact.

Next to that home was the Sardinia house. As kids we used to make a ton of noise in front of his house just to piss him off. He would come out and chase us down the street. When I was older, we began to talk and I found him to be a lot more pleasant and personable than when I was a kid. Next to Sardinia's was the Whelan home, and then my friend Jerry's house. I remembered Jerry's little dog who always barked up a storm at my setter as if to say, "You might be bigger than me, but I'll still stomp your ass!" Rory used to growl back at him as if to say back, "Watch it or I'll make you a mid-morning snack."

The famous Deluca house sat adjacent to Jerry's and there was many a night spent playing poker or other games in the basement. Sometimes in the summer we swam in his pool as well. Mike used to drive the delivery truck for one of the local supermarkets. I worked on that truck for a few years after school, trudging up and down endless flights of stairs to deliver crates of groceries to people.

Next to Mike lived Renee and her brother, Richie. I stopped there for a minute with the kids and stared at the old house now occupied by people I didn't know. Renee used to walk her dog around the same time at night that I did. On most nights when we met up during the summer, we'd spend hours talking about music and books and everything in between. I used to purposely time the dog walk with hers so we could just sit and talk. Years later, standing in front of her old house, I wondered why I never had the courage to ask her out. I guess looking back on it, I was probably scared she'd say no.

Memories of being a not-so-sure kid caused a smile to crack my lips as I remembered a friend from long ago, on a cool winter day in February.

Across the street lived Chris on the second floor. My friend, John, and his family were the superintendents of the large four apartment building complex that stood on the corner of Decatur Avenue and 204th Street. My friend Suzanne and her five siblings lived right above Leroy's' Drug store. That old building hasn't changed much over the years. The long, tan brick wall served so many purposes for all of us. We played off the wall and stickball on it. It served as the backdrop for many games of *Johnny Rides the pony*, which was a game where one team bent over and interlocked themselves making a long PONY and the other team had to run and leap onto the other teams back in an attempt to *break* the backs of the other players.

I could remember many nights coming home with a sore back and bruises, and they were all well worth it. The kids now don't play those street games anymore as in this digital age of mass media and video games, those street games have faded away into obscurity.

A funny thing about childhood memories, you can't control them once the torrential outpouring began. I looked at those old houses and remembered all those days of riding my bike and playing in the street. I could picture in my head all the parties we had at various houses and the first time I danced close with one of the girls. I felt like such an awkward geek when I did.

The blacktop was much the same as it was when I left. The kids were used to grass and concrete sidewalks in Florida and haven't seen much blacktop. I used to skate for endless hours back and forth to the park that I played roller hockey in when I was younger, all on the black top. As I looked at the cars driving past what was once my friend's father's bar, *Molly's*, I remembered the days drinking dollar drafts and hanging out with my friends.

Molly's was now a Laundromat and I suppose it was fitting. From a bar to a laundromat, smoky and dim to well lit and clean, the old building was now the complete antithesis of what it once was. Everything does indeed come full circle.

I could remember the old bars and pizza places, like 5 Brothers, Franks Deli and Volpe's Bakery. 204th Street had changed so much in the fifteen years since I left. Gone were the myriad of Irish pubs and small storefront eateries I frequented. In their place were now laundromats (and I have to say this, how many *LAUNDROMATS* are needed in a small area of space?) and many different stores and Spanish restaurants. The cars sounded the same as they cruised up and down 204th Street, the smells were different though.

Gone was the old Bainbridge Movie Theater of long ago. What was once an old fashioned movie house showing ancient style celluloid films on the big screen was now an indoor type mall. Many times in a youth, my friends and I would go to a double feature for fifty cents and spend a whole Saturday afternoon there. Long rows of broken chairs lined the aisles and there was thick, sticky, black goo on the floor that often attacked anyone who was unlucky enough to walk on it. Many days I would go home with black streaks on me from an invisible attack of the dreaded black Bainbridge Slime.

I miss watching those old movies in that theater. The goo was just part of the charm of the theater. The first real date I ever had was there. We went to the movies to see double feature with a short intermission. On Saturdays, the theater would house a lot of the neighborhood kids watching Disney films and Three Stooges shorties, all for fifty cents. Wow, can you imagine going to a movie theater now and paying fifty cents for anything much less *two* films?

I remembered how nervous I was on that first date, my palms sweaty and heart racing as if I had just run a footrace. The funny thing was if I was able to walk down what were once the aisles into the rows of chairs, I could show you where we sat. Now inside the dead theater I couldn't see anything that reminded me of what it once was. But if I close my eyes real tight and think real hard, I *could* see how it used to be. I don't remember the movies we saw, mostly because I didn't really care. The girl I was with lives in another state now and she has been happily married for almost twenty years with a family of her own. I still get a Christmas card with a photo every year.

Across from the theater sat a supermarket. Now Key Food, it was at one time The Met. I used to deliver groceries to a multitude of people almost daily after school. If I wasn't skating or playing hockey, I was in the back of the old Met van huffing and puffing up and down endless flights of stairs carrying crates of groceries to customers. We worked for tips, which on some days were very good. I think if I asked my twelve year old to do what I did at his age he wouldn't be able to. Kids now are so engrossed in today's work of super fast gratification that some of the work ethic needed for success isn't there.

My kids now are more worried about how they can level up in Pokémon and asking me to get them another game rather than actually working to earn them. If they do well in school they earn things, but it's different. Time hasn't stood still; it has changed.

I looked around the old neighborhood, absorbing the new sites and remembering the old. As I got the kids a treat for being so good, I was busy answering the plethora of questions they asked about the old neighborhood. I saw my old church and out of fear didn't walk up the hill.

I figured that if I did the roof would cave straight in on my head, after being somewhat mad at God all these years and not setting foot in a church for a long period of time.

I looked at a mural in memory of a neighborhood teen that had died tragically. I remembered a different accident in the early 90's that took the lives of six young teens. One was a kid who lived in the apartment under mine, and all these years later it seemed so surreal. I could picture very clearly the heartache and sense of tragedy the neighborhood felt for weeks and even months later.

I remembered Sunday, November 4, 1984, and the pain and sorrow it brought. I woke up early that morning for a league football game. I got to the corner to see two of my friends slumped on a car, shaking their heads in what seemed like utter shock and disbelief. Eyes red and teary, I had no idea what had happened. Then, I found out.

Shortly after 4 a.m., one of our friends was walking between two pillars under the EL across from the Terminal Bar when a drunk driver ran into him.

Apparently he died instantly. He was twenty years old.

Everyone was so distraught that we cancelled football

that Sunday. Most of us made it to the bar that afternoon, some were crying, some visibly angry, but most of us were in such a state of shock that neither anger nor tears flowed. If one tried to make sense of something like that it was a little like trying to make sense of Einstein's Theory of Relativity.

I'm not sure if there was anyone who can ever explain to me why on that day through no fault of his own, some random act happened that changed the lives of his family and took him away before his time.

I remembered that day as I walked back toward the very corner I found out about the accident. It had been almost twenty-five years now, and it seemed like yesterday when I saw him in French Charley's as he and the other guys he was with left, saying, "I'll hit ya on the field tomorrow. After I kick your ass, I'll buy you a beer."

What was so funny was that I said, "The beer is free, Pat. So is the food."

His reply was what I would have expected, "Why do think I am buying?"

We shook hands and I said, "See you at the game."

None of us saw him ever again. And I still think of him some twenty-five years after he left. I remembered playing hockey against him and the slashes across the knees from his hockey stick. I also remembered how tough he was to play against, but he was the guy you wanted on your side when the game was heated. I remembered him mostly as a guy who played hard, and in the end shook your hand and said, "Nice game. See you in Charley's."

Some things and some people just stay with you, even after they have left us.

The next days after he died were full of confusion, hurt and anger. I looked at the funeral home where so many of the neighborhood wakes took place and I remember what a colossal mess everything was that week. Hundreds of people lined up to say goodbye to him, and most of us really had no idea what to do. We milled about, some shaking our heads in disbelief. Some cried visibly and the rest comforted those who needed it.

I looked at his obviously devastated family and quietly started saying, "Please call me Mark...please..." as I stood in line to say my final good-bye. For as long as I could remember his mother never called me Mark, but always called me

Pat, her son's name. I think she always got me mixed up with another one of the kids we grew up with, or she just liked the name Patrick. I looked down at the body of a team mate, opponent, and most of all, my friend, and as I prayed silently, I listened to everyone's quiet sniffles and sobs. No one talked, or said anything. There was an astounding silence broken only by the soft sounds of muffled cries.

When I got to where his family was sitting, I saw the faces of his sisters and his best friend (and the man who married one of his sisters), their faces tear-streaked and red, and I said my condolences to his father. I hugged his mother and she said, "Mark...my Patrick...oh my poor Patrick..."

I let her go, and walked to the back of the room with my head staring at the floor. For one of the first times in my life, I had nothing to say.

Pat was buried a few days later in Woodlawn Cemetery after a crowded funeral mass at St. Brendan's Church. I visited his grave a few times and left a small pebble on the stone that marked where he now rests. Soon, I will go again, and remember my friend as I did when we were kids.

The street was alive that day as the kids and I walked past all the old haunts. I showed them the McDonalds that my mom and I worked at along with a lot of my friends. As it got later and we headed back toward the car, I could hear the old voices again, see my friends running through the streets and smell the fresh pizza from Mario's. We got back in the car and I circled the blocks one last time that day. I just silently looked.

And remembered each day of my youth with friends lost and now found again, and memories of those I haven't seen for what seems like a lifetime. I made a left turn onto Webster Avenue and drove past the old Honig's Parkway store, now a large hemodialysis center, and thought of the first ten-speed bike my dad bought me when I was twelve. Jonathan is almost thirteen now and I wish I could buy him his first ten-speed at Honig's. I wish I could, but that time is gone.

You know what? I wouldn't trade anything about where I grew up, who I grew up with, who I fought with and where I lived. I have lost contact with some, and found others, and though it has changed, this is still the place where it all began. Things always change and people move on, I have all those memories of time past. Some of them are sad, but

most of them are all good.
   I wouldn't trade them for anything.

DNR

DNR, Do Not Resuscitate. Three little letters go a long way in determining how a patient decides what they want to do in case the end of their life is near. Nurses often are approached by a patient or their family with questions regarding just what those letters mean. The first time I was asked by a patient's wife what I thought she should do regarding her husband's status, I had to think of the right thing to tell her.

Irving was a large man who walked into our hospital for elective open heart surgery to repair two leaking valves and three arterial blockages. He was in his late sixties and lived with his wife in Brooklyn, well within reach of his children and grand children. He had a large family and it was obvious when you met and spoke to him that he was the patriarch.

Coronary bypass graft surgery is what people often refer to as just plain bypass. The coronary arteries which are the arteries that feed the heart muscle itself can become blocked with fat or calcium deposits over many years. As the lumen (or opening in the artery that allows blood to flow) narrows, the blood flow to heart muscle lessens. Time passes and with arterial narrowing the risk of having blood pool behind the tightened area increases. Small clots often form, totally closing off the artery. The result is the death of heart muscle as blood flow is lost.

The resulting injury to the heart muscle causes intense pain, and the resulting heart attack is the death of the muscle itself. Sometimes patients feel angina (or *chest pain*) and there is no muscle death, but one can equate to the muscle screaming in agony for oxygen. The blockages and resulting chest pain can sometimes be *treated* (not cured) with medications. Sometimes in more serious cases a device called a stent is placed in the artery to hold it open.

Stents are placed by doctors called Interventional Cardiologists, which is a very fancy term for a doctor who fixes and opens clogged and tightened arteries without the benefit of surgery. Stents look like small springs and they are inserted and opened up in the artery. The doctor places a large

IV line in the main artery of the leg, going through the groin fold. Stents are wonderful devices that save countless people from surgery.

Sometimes stents don't work, or the arteries are so diseased that the only alternative is having the type of surgery Irving required: bypass graft surgery.

Irving was also suffering from diseased heart valves and when he was told that he needed surgery to fix both problems, he decided to have it all done at the same time so that he didn't need to have surgery twice.

Irving was a burly man, standing some six and half feet tall and close to 280 lbs. He was married to his wife for forty-five years and he had a large contingent of children and grandchildren. He walked into the hospital the night before to have pre-operative blood work and some final testing before the early morning trip to the operating room. That evening in his private room his children, wife and few of his grandchildren surrounded him in a show of love and support.

After all of the proper consents were signed, Irving had one last large meal with his family and got ready for the night. Final medications were given and all family was required to leave the unit. His wife kissed him goodbye. She said she would be waiting for him when he returned from surgery.

No surgery is ever foolproof and there are many risks associated with even the smallest of surgeries. Post operative infection is always a huge concern and the one that most people worry about. Consents are signed by the patient (or family member if the patient cannot sign), and complications are always spelled out in black and white so that everyone involved understands the risks and benefits of surgery. As a special added bonus, the last words written on the complications section are: And the possibility of *death*.

Irving left his room on a stretcher and headed for surgery early the next morning without a care in the world. His heart, which has been sick and causing him a wealth of problems, was going to be fixed and once he recovered, he would be just fine.

Except in life, not everything works out as it should.

One of the complications that can happen during open heart surgery is a stroke. A stroke is caused by one of two events in the brain. An occlusive stroke is caused by a blood clot forming, breaking off and traveling into the smaller vessels of the brain, blocking it, and causing a wide array of symptoms.

Slurred speech, weakness in the hands, confusion, vision disturbances and many others too long to list are just a few of the things that can happen as the result of a stroke. Most commonly, the patient is put on a medication regimen to control cholesterol and fats, and others to keep the blood from clumping and forming clots.

In the most severe case of stroke, a blood vessel bursts open and bleeds, and the results are usually devastating. Blood is trapped in the brain tissue causing swelling, pressure and ultimately death of healthy brain tissue. The larger the area of blood, the worse the symptoms, and the chances for recovery grow slimmer. I have seen patient's years after a devastating bleed, and it is heartbreaking to see the residual effects.

Irving had his first stoke while he was having surgery. A bleed in the right side of his brain caused left sided paralysis and profound neurological effects. When he came back to our unit he was very ill, and I was afraid that even though his heart was doing well, he as a whole wasn't. His face was drooped, his smiling ability gone and he couldn't move his left side at all. We monitored him carefully in the hope that he would begin to recover quickly.

I remember how his family, so large and supportive, was just torn apart at what had happened to him. He walked into the hospital a few days earlier, ready to have his problem fixed by one of the top heart surgeons in the country. He had a severe unexpected complication and now the prognosis for recovery was in doubt.

I left that night saddened by the turn of events, and remember hoping that by the time I came back from a three day weekend, he would have recovered some of his lost functions back. I left early the next morning on a trip to see distant family in the Albany area. It was good to get away from the monotonous grind that a large metropolitan hospital tends to be.

I came back to find Irving no longer in the coronary care unit. I was happy that he was well enough to move onto the next phase of recovery. I had no idea what had transpired while I was gone, and when I saw his wife I had a smile on my face but then I saw the look on hers. I knew something was wrong.

I asked her where Irving was and when she said the ICU, I went in quickly. There he was, lying in the bed with a respirator breathing for him. The rhythmic mechanical sound of the machine was loud and overwhelming. I looked at the bags of medications hanging on the pole, a pump carefully feeding them into him one painstaking drip at a time. I asked the nurse what had happened to him.

"He had another stroke," was the answer I got.

When I walked outside to see his wife and son I wasn't sure exactly what it was I needed to say. Words which often come easily for me, stuck in my throat and I was completely without anything productive to tell them. I asked his wife what happened, and she said that sometime Friday evening his breathing became erratic and his right side wasn't moving. A scan of his brain was done immediately and a second stroke was seen. The decision to put him on a respirator was made quickly and he was moved into the ICU. She said he was improving slowly but that she wasn't sure exactly what the doctors wanted to do.

I shook my head and said to her, "We'll wait and see if he improves. Hopefully the breathing tube can be removed and he'll recover."

When I look at that statement now, I feel kind of dumb that I even used those words, but I couldn't think of anything more than that to say. I knew the gravity of his situation and being a rather new nurse (it hadn't been a year yet), I guess I still viewed the world through rose colored glasses.

Irving improved somewhat over the course of the next week, but his movement was limited and the ability to communicate effectively and swallow food didn't return. The breathing tube in his mouth and respirator were replaced with a trachesotomy (a hole in the area of the neck just below the Adam's Apple.) and a tube into his stomach (called a PEG, and one of the things I hate as a nurse) allowed us to give him high calorie nutrition and medications. Irving had to be turned every two hours so that bedsores didn't occur and we fought a constant battle in keeping his blood pressure in check and his lungs clean of any secretions.

Day after day, time passed and it became apparent that even though we were fighting to keep Irving as well as we could, improvement had stopped. We managed to keep his skin free of breakdown, and except for a small issues, he pretty much just laid there and did nothing. His family came every single day and talked to him. They touched his hands and his face and his wife read the newspaper to him. Pictures of his grandchildren surrounded his bed.

Still Irving couldn't move nor could he speak. The only sounds from his bed was the sound of the suction machine that we used to physically remove the thick mucous his lungs made, and the electronic beeping of his heart monitor.

As devoted as the family was, the strain of seeing him in such a state began to wear on them. My job as the nurse caring for him was to keep him comfortable and stable, and to make sure that whatever I could possibly do for him and the family was done. The nurses on our unit as a whole did an excellent job in all aspects of care, and not a day went by when I didn't think we did all we could.

Sometimes it feels like a losing battle, though. I remember when I did my daily assessment dreading having to look into his eyes. Each day I looked for any sign that he could move, and none came. Daily he was turned and propped on pillows, bathed and skin care given. We made sure that when the bed was soiled (and with tube feedings such as the ones he had, he soiled it *a lot*) it was changed immediately.

I would have to look into his eyes each day I cared for him and flash a light in them to see what response I got. The more I looked, the more I knew that I was looking into a void, regardless if his pupils moved in response to my lame little light. I saw old fashioned doll's eyes, blank, and staring back at me. I knew that he wasn't going to come back and be the old Irving we had known before. I didn't need to read MRI and CAT scan results to see the obvious.

Days became weeks and weeks became months. Irving didn't improve at all, and in fact he was getting worse. The battle to keep Pneumonia at bay was being slowly lost as the opening in his neck began to breed bacteria. Antibiotics in high doses were given into his IV, and suctioning his lungs became an almost hourly routine. Each day the heart surgery residents walked in and saw him, gave a brief report and then quickly went on. His family wanted answers, and I don't think that those MD's really had any

After four months and with Irving doing worse, his wife approached me and asked if she could speak to me about something. I told her, "Of course, I'm on a break, we can speak now."

We went into the conference room and sat down. She looked bewildered and sad and obviously had a difficult topic to speak about. I simply asked her to tell me what was on her mind, and she began.

"The doctors asked me if I wanted to make Irving a DNR. And I don't know what to do. The neurologist told me that his brain will never get better and that he is slowly dying. I'm not sure what to do."

I had never spoken to anyone at all about a DNR, and I had to think carefully about what I thought was the best answer. Simply put, a DNR means do not resuscitate. If the heart stops, there is nothing that is done to restart it. There is no CPR or electric shock (defibrillation); there is no breathing support. When anything happens, as health care providers, we simply let nature take its course and let the patient expire as he should.

I sat for a minute and thought of what I should say. I started, "This is really the first time anyone has ever asked me about this, so I will ask you a few things and then you can tell me what you think."

"Okay, go ahead."

"If you and the family were sitting around the table for dinner discussing things like this and you asked Irving what it is he would want should something devastating such as this happen to him, what do you think his answer would be?"

"He wouldn't want to lie in a bed like this and not be able to anything for himself." She answered directly and fast much as I had hoped she would.

"Then I think your question is already answered. If he wouldn't want to be like this, then I would guess if given the option, he would sign the DNR paperwork so that the doctors and nurses follow his wishes."

"Do you think I should sign it?"

"I think that by answering as you did, you already know what you should do. I can't tell you to sign anything. What I can tell you is that if you know what he would want, your decision becomes easier. I think what you can do is call all your kids, go out someplace nice and talk. Talk about who

Irving was and all that he did throughout his life. Talk about the type of dad he was, and husband, and even grandfather. Remember him how he was before he came here, not as what you see now. I also think that all your family should be in on making the decision and that whatever the decision, that is best for Irving."

She nodded and said that she would call her children together and talk to them. She also asked me to call the heart surgeon so that she could talk to him. I paged him, and since they were on early evening rounds, the team would be in the unit shortly.

Irving's wife waited at the bedside with one of his daughters until the team arrived. She asked to speak to him. Though he was obviously uncomfortable and in a hurry, he did stop to talk.

She told him, "I spoke to the Neurologist about Irving and he said he won't recover anymore than he has. He is slowly getting worse and it was recommended that maybe I sign a DNR. Do you think my Irving will ever get better?"

I was completely shocked by his abrupt answer and I had to hold my tongue so hard I thought I could taste blood in my mouth as I bit down. "I fixed his heart, so as far as I am concerned, he is better. I can't predict what strokes do, but if that is what the neurologist thinks, then maybe you should."

With that he walked past her and out of the room. If silence was deafening, I was about to break it with a roar. I called my supervisor who came down into the unit. Her and I both spoke to Irving's wife.

Barbara, my boss, also spoke to the director of cardiac surgery and to the doctor himself. She wanted to speak to me about what he had said to Irving's wife but I waved her off. Though I wanted to discuss about how I explained the DNR order to his wife, I waited until the end of my shift.

Barbara thought what I said was appropriate under such circumstances. Irving's wife and daughter came back into the room and said they were meeting the rest of the family for dinner and would be back.

When she returned she asked to see the doctors and asked for the DNR order. She told us that she had sat down with her children and discussed his life, his dreams, and all the things that he had done and wanted. They decided as a family he wouldn't want to be in that bed suffering as he was, and they wanted to sign the order so that if he stopped, we didn't have to revive him.

Irving's wife signed the order and I witnessed it. She stayed for a while and held his hand and at around 11 p.m. she left to go home.

I left at 12:30 a.m. after report. Irving's breathing was more erratic and his heart rate had slowed down. I looked at him one last time and wondered if he knew he was going to die. I have often wondered just what goes through someone's head as they are actively dying. What do they see? Do they see anything? Is there really a light, or is everything just black and cold. I held his hand for a few seconds, and after a short moment of silence, I left.

Shortly before 4 a.m., Irving died. According to my colleague, he simply ceased. He took one deep breath, stopped, and then his heart shut off. It was as if he waited for his wife to let go of him and sign the order, so he knew he could go.

I didn't see his family after that. I came into work the next day and when I saw the empty bed I knew what had happened. I didn't ask any questions, but I felt as if we did what we could and when he was ready, he just stopped.

About a month or so after he died my boss came into the unit and had an envelope in her hand. She said it was addressed to the nurses and to me in particular and she wanted me to see it. I read the letter neatly handwritten by Irving's wife:

Dear Barbara, Mark and Staff:

We wanted to say thank you for the excellent care you all gave to Irving after his surgery and strokes. As a family we couldn't have asked for anything more. We think that the staff is wonderful and we wanted you all to know how much we appreciate all you did for him and us.

I was unsure of signing the order, and sitting down with Mark, who took time out from a busy day to explain to me what he thought made the decision so much easier. Thank you for taking the time out to help out a family who needed guidance. I think your supervisors should know how compassionate you were to Irving and all of us.

I wish you could have known him before he became so sick. He was a great husband, father and more so a better human being.

Thank you for being a great staff.

I wrote this about Irving not only because I remembered him, but because when I was cleaning out my files I found an old, coffee stained copy of that letter she wrote to us. I still had it, and before I threw it away (it was tattered and barely legible fifteen years later), I copied it here so I will have it forever. And so shall you, my faithful reader.

DNR. Simple letters that mean so much and can change the lives of a family very quickly. If there is anything is to be learned from this, I think it is the fact that we all as people need to consider what it is *we* want in the same situation Irving faced.

Make your wishes known, write them down, and make it legal with an attorney if you need to. I signed a health care proxy years ago after my accident and should anything ever happen to me, my family knows what I want.

I have spoken to literally hundreds of families since then, using almost the same response I gave to Irving's wife. It's easier to do now, and I find that for me, it makes the most sense when speaking to a family. The burden of deciding is much less when one considers what the person in the bed would actually want.

So, there you have it. DNR. One of the hardest decisions anyone faces.

Watch Your Speed

We all carry our own weight just like in the lyrics by Ed Roland from the song *HEAVY*, sung by Collective Soul. Some carry more and some carry less, but the plain fact of the matter is we carry the weight of everyday life on our shoulders. It is how we deal with that weight that determines the course we set for ourselves.

Anyone who tells you that they have never thought about packing it in, leaving this world (yes the operative word would be suicide, dear readers) is either a bold faced liar or completely full of shit. We all have. Each one of at one time or another has at least *thought* of it, even if it is just a fleeting instant. A mere quick thought then back to reality.

Some people, as we know, actually do kill themselves and the rest of us try to figure out what it was the caused our friend, loved one, spouse or lover to actually commit the act. In a lot of cases, there is an underlying mental illness or major depressive episode that no one was aware of. The victim simply decides that they are better off dead. They commit the act and family and friends are left behind bewildered and, in a lot of cases, angry.

The summer of 2008 was just beginning. The kids were out of school and we were spending many days poolside at our condo in Florida. The kids loved being outside swimming, and oftentimes we cooked out right beside the pool late in the afternoon when it was quiet and we could be by ourselves. We fished in the lake behind the condo and I let the kids reel in the bass and other fish I hooked for them.

On the fourth of July weekend, after refusing to help their mom move furniture into her new apartment, and after the kids were asleep, I received a message from her saying that she was leaving and never coming back.

I was left with the kids full time now. I knew by the fact that she wasn't answering messages or the phone that trying to reason with her was beyond hope. A friend and I sat down and figured out a plan of action, and we executed it a mere week later.

My friend put my children in her van and took them to

my family in New York. I filed the documents she drew up for me shortly thereafter. I waited until I knew the kids were safe in New York before I contacted their mother. I told my ex-wife that they would be there until I figured out what I was going to do. Of course, a few days later she found out I wanted full-custody and the right to move them back to New York when the police dropped the lawsuit for custody on her desk. She knew that I was serious about getting custody and moving out of Florida. If you have read this far, you know that after a lot of fighting between me and my former wife, the paperwork was drawn up and we settled before a trial, and the kids are now home with me in New York.

What you don't know is how a deep depression almost shaped the course of events differently, and how split second, impulsive decisions kept me here with them.

After the kids left and they were safely in New York, and after filing the court documents, I had a lot of time on my hands. I used that time to gather whatever evidence I needed for court, formulate a plan to get home once a judge ruled for me and gave me permission to take the kids out of state. I also thought a lot.

I thought of what kind of father I was, what kind of nurse I was, and most importantly, what kind of person I thought I was. I didn't like myself very much because I had made a series of what I thought were bad decisions, and I was ruminating on all of them.

I missed the kids despite speaking with them three or four times a day on the cell phone I got for them. I struggled with the inner demon inside of me that made my depression express itself as anger, and the anger usually won. I was mad mostly at myself for allowing things to get so out of control that I had to make the choice that I did to protect the kids from the spate of venom that was going to fly in my direction from their mother. I knew she would be angry, and I wanted the children to have a good summer away from the chaos.

I felt as if everything I touched had turned into such a colossal pile shit that each and every time I made a decision I thought it was wrong. The depression deepened, and with each day, I slipped a little further.

One Wednesday I decided to take a drive to the pier in Cocoa Beach and walk along the beach. I left in the early evening as the sun was beginning its decent in the western sky. There was a slight breeze blowing across the shore as small spindrifts whipped into the air. I could smell the fresh salty air along with a hint of decaying seaweed just barely discernable behind the odor of the beach.

The ocean has a way of making me as tranquil as I can possibly be. And although I don't consider myself a beach person, the fact that I could just walk on the beach alone in my thoughts was hard to pass up a lot of times. On most evenings, I walked there. I could watch surfers ride the waves into the shore or watch as fisherman tried to catch something good to bring home for their family.

Mostly I people watched. I liked how when the moon came up and lit the sea with a silvery light; it became more tranquil and comforting. A lot of times reflections on the water allowed me to look into myself and try to wrestle the depression demon down. This night, however, the fight was lost and I was debating whether or not I wanted to go through anything anymore.

I got into my car shortly after 10 p.m., and drove up to the hospital where I worked. I looked at the building and made my way back toward I 95 and turned to go south.

The moon was a silver coin floating in the night sky; the air was warm and crisp. My car was well tuned and doing 55...

...easy, moving at below the speed limit. I opened the sun roof and all the windows as I turned the stereo completely up... Now 60...

At 60 miles per hour, the car was like riding in a toy. I pressed the accelerator a little harder. I felt the weight of myself, my kids and the expectations of others sink into my shoulders. Tears welled up but I didn't let them fall.

70, 75, 80 and the wind was ripping through the car as the shoulder was a blur. I was driving alone and going faster. I was thinking of home, and missing my children and what would happen if...

85, 90, 95... I was thinking of how the car was responding: the engine was whirring; the highway was straight and endless and long; and no one was near. I looked for police cars and hoped one would pull me over to stop the madness inside of me. Rage and depression were steering me to go...

100, 105, 110... It's funny when you are driving that fast,

thinking about all the things you had done in your life thus far. I remembered my childhood and friends long since lost; I could see my parents and family in New York in the wind shield as the miles ripped off the odometer. The highway was a blur. I looked straight ahead and tightened my grip on the wheel. This was the fastest I had ever driven until...

115, 120, 125.... my accident in 1998. I promised myself I wouldn't have another one. I thought of the people I disappointed, those I loved and lost and how deeply saddened I was that all this had happened. I wanted to...

130, and finally, 135. My heart was pounding. I was sweating profusely despite the windows being open. The car was driving straight and true. I could see the road clearly and was thinking that if I just jerked the wheel to one side or the other I could end this mad race to nowhere. I remembered then I had a picture of the kids that was taken on my birthday earlier that year at Disney. The five of us are on Splash Mountain and you could see the fright and excitement in their eyes. I felt frightened.

If I jerked the wheel just a hair and the car lost control, how long before I felt it begin to roll? How long before it spun out of control or hit the embankment and went airborne? How would it feel if I crashed and the steering wheel hit me in the chest and pounded the life out of me? Or, how would it feel just at the point before I knew the end was there as the windshield shattered and the glass...

...I didn't know what I was doing other than driving at top speed. looked quickly in the passenger seat and for one fleeting second I saw the black angel grinning at me again. He grinned at me in 1998 when I got home, and he was smiling now. I knew what he wanted. It was my decision to make. I was confused and angry, sad and furious. I looked at him and saw a sick, twisted demonic smile that made me...

Ease up and watch the speedometer back off.

He looked at me, and I didn't pay attention. I was thinking of what the kids would think of me if I did what was on my mind. I had no one but me to rely on. I didn't dare call friends and show them what a real mess I was now. I put on a great face and smile, but all that time I hid this beast inside of me. *Now* was the opportunity to allow him to leap.

120 and still the shadow smiled. He thought he was winning, and he may have been. I was scared, but not for my-

self. I was scared of what would happen to my children, the ones I sent away to New York. What would they think if they got that phone call?

115 and the demon still wouldn't leave. I had beaten him back once, but now I wasn't feeling strong enough to try to beat him again. He sat there and looked ahead out at the road, his black hood was frightening. I could smell, almost taste the hot, fetid breath that came from beneath his dark hood. The scene was frightening and surreal, as if the path I was on was exactly what the black hooded fuck who haunts me in my dreams really wanted.

I took my foot off the accelerator, my heart was like a trip hammer, and rivers of sweat poured off of me. My shirt was soaked; my tears were hot and salty tasting. I looked at the odometer as the car was down to 90 and slowing quickly. The demon looked at me and all I said out loud was,

"Fuck you."

Not too soon after I found myself on the shoulder, stopped and waiting for the cop that never came. I had hurtled my car down a straight path to destruction, *my own*. I looked at the dark angel once again and I realized that he again, had lost. I could smell what I thought might have been a hint of sulfur in the air, but I wasn't sure if it was the water down in the drainage ditch or if it was the rubber on the tires. I was sitting in my seat, *Heavy* by Collective Soul screamed out of the speakers and I asked myself,

"What did you just do?"

The beast that had ridden with me and had *dared* me to let him win was now gone. I could still feel him there almost as if he lingered in case my dark side won. The rotten smell in the car was still there and I realized it was a mixture of my own sweat and adrenaline. Although he could have left that smell as a reminder of what still lurked inside me.

I had almost let my demons win, but in the end the visions of my children and all that they would lose and all that I would miss, snapped me back into reality. I was glad that I didn't suffer that sensation of weightlessness had the car become airborne. I didn't hear the glass shatter and see it flying toward me, nor did I feel the steering column unite with my chest in an explosion of ribs and blood.

What I felt was an incredible sense of relief, and stupidity. After I got back into the car and got off at the next exit, I picked up the phone and dialed the one person I thought could help me in a time of crisis. I called my friend and therapist, David.

I left a message that I needed to see him right away, and could he call me back in the morning.

I turned back onto the northbound section of the highway, and drove home. I did the speed limit with no visible passenger riding along with me. I got inside and took a shower because I reeked of sweat and tears and the dirt of the road, and as the hot water rolled down my back I sat on the floor of my shower and cried. Rivers of dirt and sweat and pain ran into the drain and out somewhere where it belonged. All of that spun rapidly down the pipes into some sewage treatment plant north of where I lived. I got the nastiness off of me before I laid down in a dark and empty room. I was alone, and I sat and thought about what I had almost done.

I did that because I almost took from the kids the one thing they needed more than anything. Me.

David called me in the morning and I made a bee-line for his office. He always had this unique way of spinning things just right and guiding me on the best way possible. Had I been honest and told him I actually thought of slamming the car into something at a high rate of speed, he probably would have send me straight to a doctor to get something for depression. What I did say was that I was in the midst of a crisis regarding the kids and didn't feel as if I could handle it anymore.

We sat and talked, he listened and I went on and on as I usually did. Sitting in his office at times was a painful reminder of what issues there are, what I need to solve. Other times it was a place to talk about how well things are going. I didn't want the kids to think that their dad is a weak man. I try to bury my past thoughts and faults deep so that I don't need to deal with them.

Sometimes I just become impulsive, almost like a spoiled child, and sometimes I need to just sit down and have him listen to me cry and get things out. I had made so many mistakes my pattern was to repeat most them. Having a therapist really does help whether one cares to believe it or not.

I scheduled myself for the next day as well and two sessions a week until either the kids got back from New York, or I left to join them there. My goal was to keep my eyes set straight on the prize that awaited me in New York, and to focus my energy away for summoning the self-destructive demon lurking inside of me.

I wasn't playing hockey anymore so there was no outlet for the energy that was pent up inside of me. Driving was dumb because, well, the lure of driving that car at that rate of speed was just plain insane. I knew three things. One was that no matter how badly I felt I could never actually kill myself, because, well, I had too much ahead of me to live for. That was one reason. The other was the fact that no matter how easy I thought it could be I was too chicken to actually do it.

The third thing I knew was that the kids needed me. They always had, and although I missed them like crazy and was going to fight a war in court with their mom, fighting for them was the best thing I could do. I was constantly low on money and I couldn't give them material things like I wanted, but what I could do for them was far more important in the grand scheme of things.

What I valued as being more important, was guiding them as they grow up, being what they needed me to be. If they needed a helping hand then it was my job to give it. It was also my job as Daddy to love and care for them the best as I could.

One of the things that had been so hard was feeling as if I was alone. Since my family was up north, there was no other kind of support for us in Florida. The sense of isolation I felt at times completely snuffed the life out of me. I had to face each day knowing that if I couldn't get the kids everything they needed, and maybe include something more in the deal, that I wasn't doing a good job.

Of course, having David listen to me ramble on and admit that I was indeed not Superman, SuperDad or really super anything made it easier. He allowed me to focus on the task immediately at hand, and not to allow myself to be drawn into anything that would make me spin out of control.

A few days after I almost drove into oblivion, I was fishing in the lake behind my condo, as I usually did at dusk, when the phone rang. As I spoke to each if my kids and watched the sun sink low in the western sky, the pole bent in half and line ripped off. When the seven pound bass was in my hand, I thought to myself...Watch your speed next time, when you go too fast you get into trouble.

Those lyrics from *HEAVY* still ring true today.

Weight drags you down but only when you let it. I can let the weight of life and being Daddy fall on me now because I won't let anyone else win. I can't.

You Always Remember Your First...

You always remember your first can actually mean anything, although I think that when people see a title such as this, they tend to focus on one thing only. The truth of the matter is all of us remember the first time we ever did or experienced something. I remember vividly the first time I rode a bicycle by myself at age five at the Oval. I also can see the first time I scored a goal in organized hockey as a nine-year old in CYO, which means the Catholic Youth Organization. (I can also picture scoring a ton more that year, as well.)

I remember the first time I ever slow danced at a party when I was thirteen, the first kiss I ever had, and my first date and, well, my first...child being born in November of 1996.

I think the first time you hear that you are going to be a father is exciting, shocking and, well, life-altering. I never thought I would ever meet anyone that I would marry, let alone have a child with. But I remember how it all started and how it ended with my first son lying in my hands moments after his birth.

I met my children's mother in early 1995 at orientation for my first nursing job. I was a new nurse fresh out of the wrapping paper and box, and I was a bit nervous starting my newly chosen career. I had been a pretty decent research assistant for a large investment bank for five years before deciding that I wanted to go back to school to be a nurse.

People often ask me why I chose nursing. Well, I suppose being a guy the simple answer is that I wanted to meet women. Now, although that really isn't the honest answer, it usually garners a few laughs when I say that, so most times I answer this rather dumb question with that sarcastic answer. The true answer is: I just felt as if nursing was what I was supposed to do.

I left my job and went back to school. Two and half years later, I was finished, thanks to exemptions I was able to get based on my previous degree from the same school. I passed the boards in late 1994 and soon was sitting in an orientation class at New York University Medical Center. The kids' mom was in the same class with me sitting in the front row. I took my usual last seat in the corner of the last row as I had done all through both degrees. I liked to be as inconspicuous as I could.

Most of those attending were new graduates and a few, such as the kids' mom, had experience and were going through a shortened version of the process. To be perfectly honest, I noticed her right away, but not being overly confident, (as hard as that is to believe for most of you) we didn't speak or interact in any way. Until one day about three weeks into orientation.

I was walking through the cafeteria as I always did (I am one of those very idiosyncratic people who do everything one way) and after I paid for lunch, I was walking to a table when I noticed her sitting right in line with the turnstile. I walked past her before stopping and saying, "Can anyone sit here or is it going to cost me a buck?"

She held out her hand and said, "I'll take the buck." I smiled and handed her one then I was allowed to sit. We sat and talked for a bit as we ate, easy conversation and answering simple questions such as, "Where are you from, what's your name, etc.," so when I said I knew where she was from, she looked at me and asked how a guy from the Bronx knew where her town was.

Well, the answer was easy. I told her that I played hockey in Long Beach and knew the area she lived in quite well. After we were done eating, we went to a required class and sat next to each other. As I answered the instructor's questions she gave me a look and I said, "What, you didn't know I was a genius?"

Sarcasm always wins in the end.

My birthday was a week away. I didn't see her for much of the next few days. I was just starting on the transplant unit and she was beginning her shifts in the NICU (Neonatal ICU, for premature babies). On the day of my birthday as I was standing at the nurses' station the phone rang. The clerk said, "Sure, he is standing right here."

I looked at the clerk and shrugged as if to say, "Who would call me here?" I said into the phone, "This is Mark, hello."

"Hi, this is Victoria from class, I wanted to say happy birthday."

I was shocked to say the least, so shocked in fact that I paused for a few seconds before saying, "Oh, hi. Thanks!"

The awkward silence on the other end of the phone was broken by her voice saying, "Well, I wanted to say happy birthday and see how the new job was working, I guess I'll let you go."

Before she hung up I said, "What shift are you going to be working?"

"The swing shift 4 to 12 on the 9th floor, in the NICU."

"Oh, well, me too. When you get a dinner break, let me know. Maybe I can meet you in the cafeteria. What's your unit phone number?"

She gave me the unit number and said, "Here is my home number as well, and I'm easier to reach there." And as simple as that, I had both numbers. She hung up the phone.

I have to be honest and say I never really ever had gotten many phone numbers, so I really wasn't sure when or if I should call. I did the only thing I thought I could do without looking overly anxious.

She gave me the number on Monday, and after working a double bonus shift on Friday, I went home exhausted and happy knowing I made a good amount of extra cash. I called her at home at 10 a.m. knowing she was probably out as it was Saturday morning. I went into my room and passed out cold, not really remembering much of the message I left.

I awoke out of my coma somewhere around 6:30 that evening and my mom said to me, "Some girl called and said to call her when you wake up."

"What was her name?"

"She said Victoria from work; she said she was returning your call."

I called her back at 7 p.m., and to say that she was not happy is an understatement.

The phone rang once, she answered and when I said it was Mark, she said, "Oh really?, how nice of you to call!"

"Um, is there something wrong that I don't know about?" I asked.

"*What* makes you think that?"

I answered, "Well, I worked a double bonus shift and got

the extra hundred bucks, I was pretty tired, so sorry I got back to you late."

"Well, aren't you *rich*, good for you, how are you going to spend all that extra money, Mr. Big Spender?"

Now I have to tell you, I was perplexed at this point. I called and left a message (o.k., it was pretty lame but I did call, you have to give me that), but she sounded pissed off that I actually did call her.

I said to her, "You know, I remember when we first spoke how you told me about this Japanese restaurant near you that you liked. I called to see if you wanted to go and spend my new found wealth, but if you're going to be so mad, we can forget that."

"Well, since you put it that way, I'll check to see when I am available." And with that she put the phone down. I sat there stupidly thinking to myself, *what the heck is going on here?*

About fifteen seconds passed and she came back. She said, "Well, I can meet you next Saturday any time. What do you want to do?"

"Well, how about we go to an early movie and then eat. After that if you still want to hang out we can go to Long Beach and have a drink or two."

"Fine, I'll bring the directions to my house to you on Tuesday, see you then."

Click.

I laughed to myself and thought, Well, that went just great! Let's see how next Saturday goes.

Tuesday came and at around 7 p.m. she came to my unit with 2 pages of handwritten and PRECISE directions to her parents' home in Hewlett. I told her I would call her before I left on Saturday. She left the unit and the four day wait until Saturday began.

I called her at 1:45 to say I was leaving and would be there shortly before 3 p.m. She said she would be ready and we could go straight to the movies as her parents weren't home and the movie she was thinking of started at four o'clock.

"Which movie?"

"Dolores Claiborne."

Now, I will have you know that I read the book and was a huge Stephen King fan. I said, "Great, see you in an hour."

I was dressed in jeans, a brand new pair of shoes and a casual shirt. I didn't want to overdress for a movie and dinner, but when I got to the door and she answered, I felt a bit underdressed.

She stood in the doorway, completely dressed to the nines, everything was perfectly color coordinated and matching. I kind of felt as if I needed a suit, but as I stepped into the house she quickly made me feel more comfortable as I was led into the family room. Good, I thought no parents here, at least. That was a relief.

Five minutes or so after I arrived, her parents came in the front door. They greeted me as I sat there nervously, waiting for Victoria to finish getting ready upstairs. Her father came over, shook my hand and said, "So, you're the one she's been rambling on about. It's nice to meet my new son-in-law!" And then he laughed.

I looked at him crossed eyed and laughed back, saying, "I don't know about any son-in-law, but nice to meet you sir."

"You, my friend, have been played like a fish. She has been talking about you since day one. And to think you had a few more hours before she wrote you off for good."

I wasn't following him, so I asked what he meant by that statement.

"She waited *daily* for you to call, and you never did. She told us she would give you until Saturday night to call before she forgot about you. You just made it."

Now, I knew why she was so pissed. I had to stifle a laugh and I secretly choked back a smile. It actually felt kind of good at the time, to tell you the truth.

She came downstairs and we quickly left. As we did, her dad made a gesture as if he was reeling in a fish. And it turns out he was correct in his assessment, I was nothing more than a fish.

The movie went very well then we went to the sushi place just as I told her we would. I barely ate my teriyaki chicken and she had an assorted sushi plate. I asked her if she was still mad that I had waited so long to call. She simply said, "I gave you until Saturday night, if no call by then, you were history."

"That's pretty much how your dad put it, though he calls me his son-in-law now. Kind of odd since I just met you." I laughed out loud and she looked a bit uncomfortable sitting there as I grinned.

After a nice dinner, we went to a bar in Long Beach for a drink. The bar was empty that night since it was the middle of the winter season. We sat in the back and talked some more, exchanging basic information about ourselves and work. Before we left for the night, she asked me one question,

"So, what do you want out of all of this? A relationship or is this a one-time only deal?"

I almost spit my beer about when she asked, and I quickly said, "I don't know, but this was nice, I guess we can do it again if you really want to."

We made plans for the next day and I took her home. A few short hours later I was sitting in her living room eating all my favorite appetizers as we watched a movie in her family room.

That was the start of a whirlwind romance and eventual engagement. We went fast and furious. She moved into the city in April of 1995 and soon thereafter I was spending more time in the city with her than I was at home. We became engaged in July of 1995 and took our first vacation together to Paris and London in September of that year.

I worked my nursing job and freelanced at a consulting firm so that we had the money for the wedding in May of 1996. In the middle of all the planning and saving, she came to me one night and said very matter of factly, "I have something to tell you."

"What would that be?"

"We are having a baby."

I was shocked, floored and had *no idea* what to say other than stammer out the words, "Are you sure?" She had the home test in her hand, and sure enough it showed what she had just told me; we were going to be parents.

I was happy, apprehensive and scared all at the same time. We both knew that we would keep the news to ourselves, though within a few hours our families both knew. So much for secrets, huh? Neither of us could keep one at all.

We decided that we would move into a house in Long Beach, it made perfect sense because it was close to her parents and we liked the area. It was near the rink I skated in and the area was quiet. We thought it was perfect for a new growing family.

The wedding day came on May 25, 1996, the Friday of Memorial Day weekend. We had booked the catering room on top of the St. Moritz Hotel overlooking Central Park, and it was a perfect day. We weren't of the same faith, so we decided that in the best interest of all, we would have a ceremony there first, then the reception right afterward. My parish priest married us in front of one hundred guests in a nonreligious ceremony. Shortly thereafter we had the reception.

We honeymooned in Alaska on a large cruise ship and came home to start a quite life together, and await the birth of our first child. We knew by ultrasound that it was a boy. We decided that we would call him Jonathan Benjamin, named after both of our grandfathers. So, with a name settled, we waited. And as we waited she grew, and he started to move.

Many nights as we lay sleeping I would put my hand on her belly just so I could feel him move. As a nurse, I understand everything about childbirth, but I guess feeling my child move in response to my touch completely filled me with wonder and awe.

Each day we addressed him by his name. The months peeled away quickly. His time of arrival was soon, and I was hoping for a Halloween birthday, but that came and went. Still we waited.

November 6, 1996 came and I was at work in the city. As I was driving home, my cell phone rang. It was Victoria saying that labor had started and that I needed to get home right away. I drove as fast as I could and when I arrived home she was pacing the floor wanting to go to the hospital. I asked her how far along the contractions actually were. When she said she didn't know, I waited and counted between them. Eight minutes apart. I knew we had time, but not wanting to chance anything, we grabbed the overnight bag and headed for the hospital.

When we arrived, the staff called the midwife (we chose a midwife because Victoria wanted one. Since there was *no* use in arguing, I agreed). When the first set of exams was complete, she wasn't dilated very much. We were told to go outside and walk around for a while then come back.

We walked around the hospital, then outside. Right

around the 8 minute mark we would stop as a contraction began. Neither one of us had any idea of how long we needed to walk, so we kept going until the interval for the contractions went to around seven minutes. Another exam yielded minimal dilatation. Since it was late and we were not going home, we stayed in the room with the monitor attached to her belly and watched as contractions came and went. Most of the pain was in her back. As it got later the back pain became worse. Mary, the midwife, didn't want to use an epidural as this was supposed to be natural childbirth, but as the night slipped into the early morning hours, it was obvious that pain control was becoming an issue.

I have to tell you, I went to all of the child birth classes and considered myself to be a good, well-rounded and ready coach. However, the breathing we were taught seemed to do nothing and as the pain got worse, so did her disposition.

She couldn't relax at all, which was making the pain *worse* and the progression of labor slower. Eventually, after a few hours, she was given a medication called Stadol, which managed to help her rest and allowed her to continue with labor. The funny thing is that, every six minutes, through the drug induced fog, she managed to do her breathing techniques. She couldn't answer many questions, but she remembered the breathing. At least at that point we were both able to sleep.

Labor had been going on more or less since noon on the 6th as I found out later. I called into work and told them that Jonathan was arriving and I needed off for the next few days. I figured we would both need the rest after Jonathan came.

How prophetic those words turned out to be.

The Stadol wore off and the pain wasn't any better. We called Mary again and she checked for dilatation. She was at just less than 5 cm, so Mary left the room. Victoria had a very low tolerance to pain. I cannot imagine how painful the contractions were as I have no frame of reference. I do remember Mary saying she didn't want to give her anything at that point. She left the room to go rest in the doctors' lounge.

Somewhere around 4:30 in the morning I awoke to a loud crash. When I was able to shake the sleep and cobwebs out of my head, I looked to see what the noise was.

Standing with the monitor still on her belly and half

crazed with pain was Victoria holding a folding chair. When I asked what she was doing she said, "If I don't get something *NOW, SOMEONE* is getting *SMACKED* with this."

I got her back into the bed and went outside to the nurses' station to speak to the doctor on call. Victoria actually knew both Mary and the doctor from her previous work at that hospital. When he came into look at her he asked her ONE question:

"Do you want an epidural?"

"*YES!*"

"So, have them come so we can move on here." And he left the room. Anesthesia came into the room, gave her the epidural and she lay back and tried to relax. The decision to use a medicine to induce labor was made, as well. Within a few minutes of the medication starting, the contractions came in waves.

Once she was relaxed and dilatated, the pushing began. I had never seen a live child birth. I was filled with excitement and wonder as I watched my son being born.

I didn't expect it to be like a television show, and it really wasn't. I saw the top of his head crown and it was then I realized that this was real. I was about to see the person I waited my *whole* life to see. My son was coming and he was coming fast.

She was pushing and crying and I could see the intensity in her eyes as she concentrated and focused. His head was coming! I could see his hair and with each effort he was a little closer to being real.

Soon, with a mighty push, I could see his face! White with a waxy substance and purple from no breaths yet, I looked at my son's face for the first time and I felt an incredible sense of love and some fright. I was waiting for the rest of his body to come out. I wanted to see him and hold him and protect him as *DADDY* was supposed to.

Another push and his shoulders were in view. He was coming and she was exhausted. I told her to push as hard as she could so that she could see the child she had been waiting for. I looked down and in a rush of fluid and blood and with one mighty roar from his mother, Jonathan slid into the waiting hands of the midwife and me.

She quickly cleaned his nose and mouth and the little purple figure in her arms started screaming. As he did, his color changed from that deathly purple into a wonderful shade of pink.

My son was here. And he was beautiful.

I was able to cut the cord and we both held him together. That day changed my whole life. In one final effort and push from his mother, he came into the world on November 7, 1996.

You *never* forget your first. And I haven't ever forgotten my second, or my third...and not my fourth, either. Each one of my children was born into my waiting hands. It is an experience that will remain with me forever.

Jonathan is twelve now. I can close my eyes and see his wrinkled, purplish face as he came into this great, big, scary world we live in. I was ecstatic when he came to us on his very first day, and not a day goes by that I don't remember what a gift all the kids are.

He was and is always my first. You *never* forget that. Never.

LOOK AT ME, DADDY

Looking back over the years at all of the things that have come and gone, I think that watching the kids do something that gave them a sense of accomplishment has made me happiest. Learning new words, drawing a picture or telling me something that made them proud of themselves was always something that I enjoyed experiencing.

As the kids birthdays arrived during the latter portion of 2007 and into 2008, I was able to save enough money so that each one could pick out a brand new bicycle. Jonathan's birthday came first in early November of 2007. When it was time, he picked out the one he wanted and helped me push it to the register so that we could pay for it. Once that was done, we took it to the car and brought it home. He was able to ride it in the parking lot of our condo development.

Before I began renting the condo in November of 2006, we had lived in a large, newly built five bedroom, three bathroom home in Rockledge, Florida. We had a large backyard (soon replaced by a large pool and spa, all screened in to keep the critters out) and a three car garage that allowed for the storage of a variety of riding toys. Among them was a large, two wheeled kick scooter that my mother had purchased on one of her infrequent trips to see us.

The kids had a lot of problems trying to learn to ride their bikes without training wheels. The two older ones would get frustrated and scared as we tried to help them learn the intricacies of balancing themselves on two wheels. The little boys loved taking turns on the large battery operated car we had purchased, and Jon and Julia rode bikes with training wheels up and down the sidewalk for hours.

No matter how hard we tried to help them, they couldn't balance right and got scared each time the bike would tilt to the side. I think the fear of scraping themselves on the concrete or the mechanics of riding the bike were the fears that they had most. I figured eventually learning to balance the bike would just come to them.

The house we had built faced a two acre nature preserve that was home to a plethora of wildlife. Ibis, Cormorant,

Sandhill cranes and other types of waterfowl gathered in the early morning and at dusk to feed on the overabundance of insects and frogs that inhabited the wetland. With all of the birds around there was never a mosquito problem, which was a huge relief.

Every so often at night we would hear a huge splash and the occasional *thud* above the song of the insects and frogs. Although I only saw a glimpse one morning at the large alligator that made his home there as he walked across my lawn, I was able to hear the aftereffects of whatever meal he picked off from the many choices on the dinner menu. There was once a flock of ducks that lived there for a while. I think one by one they became a meal for the large reptile.

After weeks of trying to get the kids onto a two wheeler and watching how frustrated and scared they got trying to balance themselves, I was about ready to throw in the towel. I looked for alternatives for them. Without realizing it, a good one sat on a hook in the garage.

That scooter was like a two wheeled skateboard. I thought that if they could balance and steer the scooter, then riding a bike would just come naturally. I took the scooter down and had Jonathan come over to try to see how he would do riding it rather than the training wheeled bike he was on. At first, his apprehension and fear of falling got the best of him. But after a little persuasion, he got on the scooter and I ran with him as he tried to steer. His balance was off, but, all-in-all, I could see that he would soon be able to ride the scooter. Then the bike would soon follow.

I ran along side of him for a bit, but eventually I gave into my own sense of fear of falling and let him ride. He fell quite a few times, but he managed not get angry at himself. He would get right back on and try again.

The routine of riding and balancing continued for a few short days. When I saw how well he had progressed, I knew that it was a matter of time before he began to master it. He still pitched the scooter to the side each time he felt it teeter to one side or the other. All I could offer were words of encouragement and the standard, "Keep going, you're doing great!" He tried as hard as he could, and met with the same frustration day after day, but he pressed onward.

The luxury of having a yard and a relatively quiet street allowed the kids to run around outside and play as much as possible. Each day brought a new set of challenges and rounds of practice on the scooter. One day, I noticed that as Jonathan was pushing the scooter, he was holding on and steering much better. He was balancing and riding, and it was if he had no idea he was doing it.

That was just the opening I needed to encourage him to try the bike again. I worked nights, and on those nights I worked I often slept for a few hours in the afternoon, so I hadn't been out watching the kids play. I had a feeling that if I could convince Jon to try the bike, the great scooter experiment would be a success.

I took his bike out of the garage and quickly removed the clunky training wheels from it before I called him over. He put the scooter down and I told him I thought he should try to ride the bike now. I thought he would do great and was now ready.

Of course, he was scared. But I told him I wouldn't let go and would run with him until he was riding. He sat on the saddle and started to pedal as I held the back of the seat. I could tell right away that as soon as I let the seat go he would be riding it solo. I ran and yelled encouragement at him. As I was doing so, I let go.

Off he went down the street, not even realizing I was behind him, watching him meander down the street all by himself! I was so proud of him. He turned the bike around and came back all excited, as he jumped off and yelled, "Daddy, I *did it!*" I grabbed him and told him how great he was and to keep riding.

He did. Each turn yielded more confidence and speed and daring. He became quite an accomplished rider quickly, he has been ever since.

As soon as he accomplished riding his bike, I immediately got Julia on and doing the same things he did. Julia turned out to be a challenge, as well. Her coordination and balance for a time was worse that Jon's. As she gained control and confidence steering the scooter became easier for her. A few weeks later it was her turn for me to hold the seat as she pedaled her two-wheeler for the first time.

After weeks and weeks of practice and trying as hard as they could, both Jon and Julia had gotten past their initial fears and were riding up and down the block as proud of themselves as they could be.

A few months after they learned to ride, I was busy packing up the remainder of the house because we were getting ready to move out after the sale of the house. Our marriage had completely fallen apart and I was in danger of having to go into foreclosure because I was unable to make enough money on my own to keep the house. I held on as long as I could. Each day the depression that I had became heavier and more entrenched inside of me.

My work became affected and I wound up leaving Parrish Medical Center because I wasn't able to handle the pressures of working nights and dealing with a total disaster at home. My boss at the time, Pam, who is still to this day my biggest supporter in Florida, asked me to get myself straightened out before I could come back and work in the hospital. It was the first time in my life that anything of the sort had ever happened to me, and although I knew it wasn't personal, it hurt me deeply.

It also made me come back months later stronger. I was the nurse she needed me to be. Not being there allowed me to a take a day shift job at a competing hospital for a year, where I was able to spend more time with the kids and try to stabilize things as best I could. When I asked Pam if I could work directly for the hospital as opposed to through my agency, she hired me immediately. When I left a year later, it was the hardest time I ever had leaving a job.

How do you thank someone for seeing the problem and allowing you to return to a job you liked before, and caring enough to see that your children are always cared for and safe?

In a way, I think I just did.

That old scooter never made it to the condo complex I rented. The tires were old and warped, and I basically had no room to store it. I donated it to a Christian church not far from me, and I decided not to buy a smaller one. When the kids went to their mom's house for her time on weekends, they rode their bicycles there. The little boys continued their tradition of using the battery operated car.

For the most part, the kids were with me and during the week it became a routine of driving back and forth to school, homework for the four of them then some down time before bed. I didn't have much of an opportunity to work with the little boys on how to ride a two wheeler, and I didn't give it a lot of thought. As their August birthdays arrived in 2008, they were in New York City while I fought for full custody.

When the kids came back from New York and school began, I had them full time until mid September when their mom decided she wanted them on weekends again. The kids wanted to see her, so without a lot of fanfare, we slipped back into the routine of the kids at her house on weekends. We weren't speaking at all, and the exchanges were no more than the kids saying goodbye to either of us as they transferred houses.

One night in late September I arrived in the evening to pick the kids up when I noticed Alex riding a small razor scooter. He was zipping along at a fast pace, perfectly balancing himself and steering the scooter around a small course he had outlined in chalk.

After all the things said about Alex and his developmental problems, I was amazed that he drew out a path as he did. I shouldn't be because he pretty much amazes me daily. I asked the kids to get in the car. Once they were done with goodbyes to their mom and her new husband, I took them home thinking that the next day I was going to see how Alex did on his bicycle. I had purchased two bikes with trainers a month before, and the little boys rode them in the parking lot at the condo complex.

The long, winding parking lot at our place had a lot of room for the kids to ride. There was a path that wrapped around the grounds. On some days we all rode along that path then took ourselves outside to the municipal park that was across from where we lived. Oftentimes, the little boys would complain that it was too far to ride, but my ulterior motive was to have them burn off excess energy and be tired so that they could sleep at night. The training wheels made it bit harder for them to ride, and they didn't like the longer days we spent on the path.

I took the bikes out of the small storage unit I had rented and had the kids ride to the front of our building. I told Alex that I thought it was time to take the training wheels off. All he said was, "Okay dad."

I unscrewed them and put a helmet on his head. I have a video camera in my phone in case I see something worth filming, so I set the camera to record.

I took my usual position behind him and held the seat.

We ran together as the other three watched us go. I was telling him to keep pedaling, and as I let the seat go, something wonderful happened.

My little boy, the one who no one said could be normal, rode his bike alone. He had problems coordinating the handle bars and braking, but he was pedaling! I was so excited that when I was yelling, "You're doing it!" he turned to look at me and promptly crashed into the curb.

No matter though; he did it. I helped him get back on the bike and he began his second ride alone with a better handle on control. I filmed everything. After I watched him and heard him say, *"Daddy, look at me! I'm riding!"* I beamed with pride and cried with enjoyment.

I called everyone. My excitement was such that I couldn't even speak that long. I watched in wonder as my son, the one all the experts said was mentally handicapped and wouldn't be able to do many of the things other kids do, trumped them all by learning to ride a bicycle. And he did it without even realizing he was learning.

That Razor scooter and all those times he rode in front of his mom's house trained his body to coordinate and balance.

My son. He fills me with wonder every single day. He accomplished what many people may consider something small, but to us, it wasn't.

Hearing him say *"Daddy, look at me"* was one of the proudest moments of his young life. And as the days pass us by here in New York, I wonder just what those words will mean the next time. Pride and accomplishment for a child no one believed in except his parents is something no one can ever replace.

The sky truly is the limit.

Why is the Closet Closed?

We all have fears. Some of them are completely normal, such as the fear of falling or the fear of death. Some of them can be overwhelming and manifest themselves in phobias, such as the fear of the number thirteen or the fear of spiders. I have my own irrational fear, and it is why I keep my closet door closed.

When I was a kid and we lived in a small one bedroom apartment in the Bronx, my parents, my sister and I all slept in the same room. My sister had the bottom bunk and I slept on the top, in full view of the small closet in the corner of the room. Many nights before I finally drifted behind the wall of sleep, I would look into that closet and see the eyes staring back at me. I could hear the scratching and the laughter, and I didn't know if it was in my head, or it came from the closet itself.

I remember as a forth grader a notice was sent out to parents that said a gray car with two men inside was trying to lure children to a party. We were warned *not* to engage the men, or to get into the car. If a stranger approached us, we were to call for an adult or run away.

The day the gray car approached us as we were playing, is probably the principal reason why I fear what I find to be the scariest thing in the world. I still have that irrational fear even as a semi rational forty-four year old father of four.

One day I was in the mall with all of my kids, I was pushing the double stroller along and Jon and Julia were walking beside me. I had taken the kids to buy shoes, and being pretty frugal, I usually took them to the discount shoe place where I often found a two for one sale or buy one pair and get 50% of a second pair. Buying shoes for one kid can be a chore. Having all four of them at the same time was just plain crazy. I often got looks from other shoppers as the kids would scream, *"Daddy, I want this,"* or, *"Can I get these shoes please?"* In most instances, I tried to keep them calm. Sometimes it was damned near impossible.

We visited various stores that day. After I bought a few soft, hot pretzels and lemonade (which I must say, whenever

I go to a mall that is the one place I always stop) we headed toward the food court as the kids wanted something more substantial.

The mall wasn't overly crowded and the Food Court was rather empty. It was sunny and warm outside, and the sun shone through the glass roof, brightening up the whole area. I knew the kids always gravitated toward the pizza stand while I preferred Chik-Fil-A. I went to get my usual #1 combo (I like the chicken sandwiches, but the cow ads are frigging hilarious.), then I ordered slices of pizza for each of my kids and I sat down with the four of them. Out of the corner of my eye I noticed two figures going table to table and handing out cards and balloons. My heart started going faster and the kids got excited.

Fucking great, I thought, just what I need: *clowns*.

Now I know as a faithful reader you must be asking yourself, "What is the deal with clowns?" I don't know if I have a rational answer other than to say I think that under all make-up lurks someone who is hiding something. I think of the famous Pennywise from the novel IT and remember what a twisted, sick, evil figure he was. And, he was a clown. John Wayne Gacy, Jr., the mass murderer often is pictured in clown face. I see movies titled *Killer Klownz from Outer Space* and think that they are evil, demented characters. Clowns have scared me since I was a child. Even now at forty-four years of age, I still close my closet door in case there is one lurking in the shadows. Because that is what evil clowns do; they lurk in the shadows and pounce.

My kids think it is hilarious that Daddy fears what they consider to be happy and carefree characters. The reality is I do not think it is funny at all. I see a clown and my insides turn over. I feel a sense of urgency and a need to flee the room. I can't look at them, talk to them nor do I even want to be at a kid's show where there is a clown. I started closing my closet door many years ago because I always thought that the threat of clowns hiding in there and jumping out at me was always a possibility.

As we sat there, the two clowns waved at the kids and moved to come over. I started to pack up as fast as I could. After they got to the table the kids were chatting away and asking for animal balloons. One of the clowns was a lady who spoke in a soft voice to the kids. She could see that I wasn't too happy that they were there.

I was trying my best *not* to be rude or inconsiderate in front of the children, but she could see how much of a hurry I was in. She asked if there was something wrong. I quickly said, "Nothing other than we are leaving, Miss. Thanks."

"Can we leave a business card? We do parties and special events for kids."

"No, thanks, we really need to go."

She gave me a somewhat astonished look as I hurriedly took the two older ones by the hand and pushed the stroller through the maze of kids surrounding the two clowns.

My heart was beating fast and I was happy to get away. Just in the nick of time, too.

The kids constantly asked me why I was in such a hurry to leave. I told them that Daddy is not a fan of clowns and that, as funny as it sounds, he is afraid of them. Jon asked if it was like being afraid of big bugs. My answer was simply that clowns to me were worse and I don't like being around them.

"That's weird, Daddy. Clowns are nice!"

I thought to myself, *no son they aren't. They appear that way, but to me they aren't. Why do you think I keep the closet door closed?*

I can trace that fear back to the one day my friends and I were playing a game called Skully (a board is drawn, or in this case, painted on the sidewalk) in which each of the players has a bottle cap usually filled with molten crayon or candle wax. The object of the game is to go from numbered box to numbered box and at the end become a killer. Once the player becomes a killer, he hits his bottle cap into his opponents three times effectively killing them for the game. We used to have games that had six or seven guys and lasted hours.

As we sat in the street playing, a gray car pulled up and stopped. Inside were two men in clown face and they started talking to us. Each of us had been warned a few days before about the car, but the men were persistent.

They offered a party at an apartment on the other side of the parkway complete with cake, music and fun. We kept saying, "No, thanks", but they persisted anyway. Finally, after two or three minutes of getting nowhere with us, and after one of my friends ran to get his dad, the car sped up the street. One thing though, my friend and I got a copy of their plate number.

Soon after the incident a police car came and the officers asked us a battery of questions. What kind of car? What color? What did they say? How are they dressed? Well guys, they were dressed like clowns and NOW I had absolutely NO desire to ever see one again. I used to watch reruns of *Bozo the Clown* on an old black and white set in my bedroom. That ceased the day those two men tried to get me and my friends into a car with them.

When the police were done asking questions they asked if we had anything else to tell them. My friend Rob said, "Well, me and Mark got the license plate. Is that good enough?" When the cop asked us why we didn't tell them that first, the answer I gave was simple, "You didn't *ask*, Sir."

Off sped the cop car up the street, and back we went to our Skully game.

That night I closed the closet door for the first time because I saw those clown faces in the dark. I stayed awake all night in fear.

The following Monday while we were in school the morning announcement was filled with the usual Monday morning fodder except for an extra tidbit. "The men in the gray car were arrested yesterday after the police were able to trace them using information given to them by some students here."

If the television show the *Worlds Dumbest Criminals* existed back then, those two idiots would be on television in *prime time*. The moron who drove the car actually used his own plate and never thought any kid was smart enough to take the number down.

And it turns out idiot number one, the driver, was wrong!

My kids and I got home as it was getting dark. I made sure that when they went to bed, all of the closet doors were closed. My now ex wife thought it was the stupidest thing she had ever heard; a grown man running out of the mall in fear of two people dressed as clowns, and making sure all of the closets were closed again.

As dumb as it sounds, it had to be done because I can still see and hear those two clowns from when I was a kid. At night when I am alone, I can hear the breathing of the monster waiting to come out of the closet. As long as the door is closed we are all safe.

Hiding my head under the blankets doesn't work anymore.

The End?

What is The End? I'm not exactly sure how to answer that question because right now there really isn't an end, per se. The kids are growing in leaps and bounds, and since the big, dramatic move in December, each of them has done nothing short of prosper and done better than I could have expected. As hard as moving away from Florida and from their mother has been, they have thrived here in New York in an environment of family, friends, structure, and support.

So what happens now, dear reader? I'm sure that the million dollar question is, "What is left, and what stories did you leave out?" Well, I suppose if I revealed all, then there wouldn't be enough to give you next time. Let's leave it at this: there is so much more to say.

Raising children isn't easy even with two parents. I don't judge success in parenting on how well a child does in a career after he has been raised. What I look for is respect and love of others and how complete the child is as an adult to gauge how successful parents are. I don't consider myself to be anything more than the daddy to my kids. Years from now I hope someone can say that I did a halfway decent job, and not a half-assed one.

I have a wealth of issues that any one of my faithful readers can recognize in just about anything I write. I have battled through bouts of depression so severe that I felt as if I was better off in a box somewhere. The only thing that pulled me out was the overwhelming responsibility I have as a dad. I love my kids more than myself, and if it weren't for them, where I would be now is debatable.

I have scared myself on more than one occasion, and have placed a tremendous burden on people around me as I battle that inner demon that sits somewhere deep inside of me. Writing helps, as does talking things out. But when one internalizes everything it creates this volcano that stands on the edge of erupting at any time.

I think being a nurse adds to the stress level, and although I have this incredible capacity to care for others, I have an equally hard time caring for myself. That is an issue

I work on, and will continue to do so. I hope in the end, the people who were caught in the tidal waves I was a part of can be forgiving of the repeated mistakes that were made. My kids will realize one day that all Daddy was was a person who gave himself to others before he gave to himself; that he made for a very sad person at times. I ask that once they realize who Daddy is and what he did for them as a person, that in the end, everything turns out as good as it could have.

I hope that the clowns stay away for good and that all of you do well in your own lives. I look forward to the meeting each and every reader and thanking you in person. I anxiously await each day as my children take one step closer to adulthood. For myself, I hope that I do a successful enough job and the threat of the demon of depression finally stays in his box.

I urge anyone with a child like my Alex to be aware of anything that might explain the reason why they are diagnosed as Autistic. I can state from my own experience that everything is not clear cut and as black and white as it seems. I know what happened to Alex, and I think as a responsible person I should state to all of you with children such as him to look at the records if your child was jaundiced. There is a direct correlation between high counts and brain damage, so if you have any doubt, research the subject. I have, and no matter what anyone says, doctors and experts can be wrong.

As a parent it is my job to be the best for my kids, and as a responsible health provider, I urge you to not take any diagnosis of Autism lying down, to consider all facts before a blanket diagnosis is given.

How does a fledging author such as me thank a tireless reader? I don't think I adequately can. Words on a page or spoken out loud can never thank anyone enough for taking the time to read the words I wrote, and for the encouragement given to me when I thought I couldn't do it.

So, thank you, tireless and dear reader, for taking the time to read the perspective of a daddy and a nurse. For those who know the real me, thank you for allowing me the opportunity to include you in these little trips I took.

I also know that when I look back at writing all of this, the next chapters I give will be hopeful and bright and re-

freshing to all of you.
   Until we meet again...

About the Author

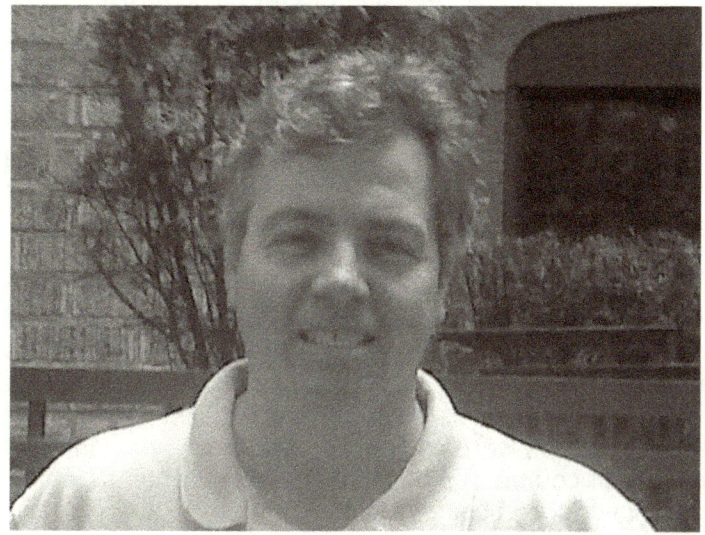

Photo by Alex McGrath

Mark McGrath is a single father of four children currently residing in Bayside, New York. Born and raised in the Bronx, he attended St Brendan School and moved on to Cardinal Spellman High School, graduating with the famed class of 1983.

He worked as a research librarian assistant for Lehman Brothers in the late 1980's and early 1990's while he attended Lehman College in the Bronx. Graduating with a Bachelor of Arts in Economics in 1989, he quickly changed course and began nursing school in 1991. He again attended Lehman College and while in school worked for Booz Allen and Hamilton and AT Kearny in New York City as a consultant researcher.

He graduated Cum Laude from Lehman's nursing program in May of 1994 and passed the Boards in September of that year to become a Registered Nurse. New York University Medical Center was his destination soon after where he worked on the liver and kidney transplant unit starting in 1995.

His first son, Jonathan, was born in 1996, and soon after he relocated to Ronkonkoma, New York, taking a job at Stony Brook University Medical Center as an assistant to the Nurse Manager running the middle shift. After suffering injuries in a car accident in 1998, he moved on to become an IV Nurse Educator in Farmingdale, teaching IV skills to other nurses, and seeing home care clients.

He relocated to Florida in October of 2001 and worked for a nursing agency that sent him to various hospitals as a traveling RN. He took his last permanent job in Florida in 2007 at Parrish Medical Center in Titusville.

After gaining custody of his four children in October of 2008, he moved back to New York to start over again. He currently works as a home care IV specialty nurse and still teaches nurses IV skills.

In his spare time he enjoys going out and spending time with his children, watching his favorite teams win (Jets, Yankees and of course, his beloved Rangers), and has recently began playing ice hockey again.

www.ingramcontent.com/pod-product-compliance
Lightning Source LLC
Chambersburg PA
CBHW020002050426
42450CB00005B/281

And we all continued to watch Rico.

Still he struggled, and his breathing remained in the high forties. His daughters were each holding an arm and his wife was stroking his face telling him it was all okay now, that they would be fine and to please go to wherever he needed to go. They all told him to let go, that the family loved him and would miss him, but that his suffering needed to end. His breathing came in short pants, much as a winded athlete breathes after a long race or shift of ice time on a hockey rink (something yours truly can personally relate to).

I listened silently and struggled with the scene myself as it was heart rendering and touching to witness. I thought to myself how lucky he was to have a family who loved him so much that they *wanted* him to die so that the pain and illness he was suffering would finally come to an end. The girls were begging Daddy to please let go and stop suffering. The sobs coming from them were unbearable for me to hear.

I watched intensely as another half hour rolled past and Rico continued to writhe and moan. As soon as I was able, I increased the drop rate to eight mg an hour and went about monitoring his progress. His respiration rate dropped from the mid fifties to around forty. But even though the rate had dropped, he still was uncomfortable and was extremely restless.

I called Barbara when I increased the rate and asked her to please come speak with me on my dinner break. She told me she would be there shortly and to meet her in the conference room. I told her I would and got myself ready to leave for a well deserved half hour break.

I quickly gave my relief nurse an overview of what was going on and told her that I would change the drip rate if needed when I came back. Both of Rico's daughters had left to get something to eat themselves and his wife had her head on his hand in what seemed to be a prayer vigil.

I met Barbara in the conference room and gave her the latest news on how he was doing. She knew I was still struggling with things and she sat listening *again* about how I felt. I told her that I felt I was contributing to his death and that I was having an issue increasing the drip to 16 mg.

What she said to me made a profound difference in how I

have approached life and death since that day in the ICU. She told me to put myself in Rico's place, and asked what would I want?

"Not to be in pain, that's for sure", was the first thing I said.

"Mark, he is terminal. You are smart enough to understand what's happening and know that nothing more can be done. The family wants his suffering to stop. Whether he dies now, five minutes from now or five hours from now, don't you think that the best thing is be humane and make him as comfortable as you can? You can't kill someone with humanity, Mark. What you can do is treat him as best as you can given what you know, and make the last hours as pain free and comfortable as humanly possible. You need to increase the drip and not worry about *how* things look. Remember that you are the nurse in charge of making sure he is getting what he needs to be comfortable and pain free. If that was you there, what would you want your family to tell me to do?"

As I listened to her words, I realized that she was right. Both rules applied here: he was one of those patients who got sicker and was going to die, and nothing I knew or did would ever change the fact that he was going to die. So, I did what I would want someone to do for me in my time of dying, in pain, and suffering unbearably.

I went back into the ICU and turned the drip rate to 16 mg.